Emergency Triage

Telephone triage and advice

Emergency Triage

Telephone triage and advice

Manchester Triage Group

EDITED BY

Janet Marsden

Mark Newton

Jill Windle

Kevin Mackway-Jones

FIRST EDITION

(VERSION 1.7)

BMJ|Books

WILEY Blackwell

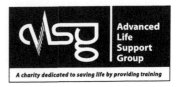

This edition first published 2016 © 2016 by John Wiley & Sons, Ltd. This version updated 2023 (Version 1.7)

Registered Office
John Wiley & Sons, Ltd, The Atrium, Southern Gate, Chichester, West Sussex, PO19 8SQ, UK

Editorial Offices
9600 Garsington Road, Oxford, OX4 2DQ, UK
1606 Golden Aspen Drive, Suites 103 and 104, Ames, Iowa 50010, USA

For details of our global editorial offices, for customer services and for information about how to
apply for permission to reuse the copyright material in this book please see our website
at www.wiley.com/wiley-blackwell

The right of the author to be identified as the author of this work has been asserted in accordance with the UK
Copyright, Designs and Patents Act 1988.

Library of Congress Cataloging-in-Publication Data

Emergency triage (Manchester Triage Group)
Emergency triage : telephone triage and advice / Manchester Triage Group ; edited by Janet Marsden,
    Mark Newton, Jill Windle, Kevin Mackway-Jones. – First edition.
        p. ; cm.
    Includes index.
    ISBN 978-1-118-36938-8 (pbk.)
I. Marsden, Janet, editor.   II. Newton, Mark, 1963– , editor.   III. Windle, Jill, editor.   IV. Mackway-Jones,
Kevin, editor.   V. Manchester Triage Group, issuing body.   VI. Title.
[DNLM: 1. Triage–methods.   2. Emergency Service, Hospital.   3. Telephone.   WX 215]
    RA975.5.E5
    362.18–dc23
                                        2015007951

A catalogue record for this book is available from the British Library.

Wiley also publishes its books in a variety of electronic formats. Some content that appears in print may not be
available in electronic books.

Set in 9/12pt Meridien by SPi Global, Pondicherry, India
Printed and bound by CPI Group (UK) Ltd, Croydon, CR0 4YY
C9781118369388_091023

Contents

Editors

Janet Marsden, Professor of Ophthalmology and Emergency Care, Director – Centre for Effective Emergency Care, Manchester Metropolitan University.

Mark Newton Head of Service/Consultant Paramedic responsible for Urgent Care. North West Ambulance Service NHS Trust

Jill Windle, Lecturer Practitioner in Emergency Nursing, Salford Royal Hospitals NHS Foundation Trust and University of Salford.

Kevin Mackway-Jones, Consultant Emergency Physician – the Manchester Royal Infirmary and the Royal Manchester Children's Hospital, Medical Director – North West Ambulance Service, Honorary Civilian Consultant Advisor in Emergency Medicine to the British Army, Professor of Emergency Medicine – Centre for Effective Emergency Care, Manchester Metropolitan University.

Acknowledgements

The editors would like to thank all those in the North West Ambulance Service who have contributed their time and expertise to this project and in particular to Stephanie Allmark and Stephen Scholes whose contribution and support remains absolutely invaluable.

Members of the Original Manchester Triage Group

Kassim Ali, Consultant in Emergency Medicine

Simon Brown, Senior Emergency Nurse

Helen Fiveash, Senior Emergency Nurse

Julie Flaherty, Senior Paediatric Emergency Nurse

Stephanie Gibson, Senior Emergency Nurse

Chris Lloyd, Senior Emergency Nurse

Kevin Mackway-Jones, Consultant in Emergency Medicine

Sue McLaughlin, Senior Paediatric Emergency Nurse

Janet Marsden, Senior Ophthalmic Emergency Nurse

Rosemary Morton, Consultant in Emergency Medicine

Karen Orry, Senior Emergency Nurse

Barbara Phillips, Consultant in Paediatric Emergency Medicine

Phil Randall, Consultant in Emergency Medicine

Joanne Royle, Senior Emergency Nurse

Brendan Ryan, Consultant in Emergency Medicine

Ian Sammy, Consultant in Emergency Medicine

Steve Southworth, Consultant in Emergency Medicine

Debbie Stevenson, Senior Emergency Nurse

Claire Summers, Consultant in Emergency Medicine

Jill Windle, Lecturer and Practitioner in Emergency Nursing

International Reference Group

Austria
Stefan Kovacevic
Andreas Lueger
Willibald Pateter

Brazil
Welfane Cordeiro
Maria do Carmos Rausch
Bárbara Torres

Germany
Joerg Krey
Heinzpeter Moecke
Peter Niebuhr

Mexico
Alfredo Tanaka Chavez
Elizabeth Hernandez Delgadillo
Noe Arellano Hernandez

Norway
Grethe Doelbakken
Endre Sandvik
Germar Schneider

Portugal
Paulo Freitas
Antonio Marques
Angela Valenca

Spain
Gabriel Redondo Torres
Juan Carlos Medina Álvarez
Gema García Riestra

Preface

It is now 20 years since a group of senior emergency physicians and emergency nurses first met to consider solutions to the muddle that was triage in Manchester, UK. We had no expectation that the solution to our local problems would be robust enough (and timely enough) to become the triage solution for the whole United Kingdom. Never in our wildest dreams did we imagine that the Manchester Triage System (MTS) would be generic enough to be adopted around the world. Much to our surprise, however, both of these fantastic ideas came about, and the MTS continues to be used in many languages to triage tens of millions of Emergency Department attenders each year.

Clinical decisions made by telephone have always been an area of concern for clinicians because not only is the patient not present and it may be difficult to obtain correct information but many of the tools and indicators that we use for decision making are simply not available. It is therefore an inherently more risky process than face-to-face triage.

Quite early on in the implementation of MTS in Manchester, departments began to use a simplified version as a structure for telephone conversations. This was superseded by national algorithm-based telephone helplines and its use in the Emergency Department diminished.

Our colleagues in the Greater Manchester Ambulance Service (GMAS) felt that there was a gap in their resources for undertaking telephone decision making. We have discussed ways of developing tools based on the MTS, with its significant evidence base and good safety record which would embed safety and quality into their telephone decision systems.

A huge amount of work has been done by the now North West Ambulance Service (NWAS) along with MTS to test and audit a robust Telephone Triage tool. It has also been piloted in diverse settings, with ambulance services in the Azores and New Zealand, as well as other services in the United Kingdom using it for the whole or part of their day to day work. It has been tested and refined and has a superb audit trail and safety record associated with it.

The basic principles that drive the MTS (recognition of the presentation and reductive discriminator identification) are unchanging – but changes have been made to reflect the difficulties of assessment by telephone. The outcomes of decisions are condensed into 'face-to-face now', 'face-to-face soon' and 'face-to-face later' with a self-care outcome. Information and advice is suggested alongside every outcome. The advice ranges from life-saving interventions which can be carried out until health care arrives, to self-care advice.

We recognise the diversity of health care settings and the need for appropriate information and advice; therefore, the information and advice sections of the Telephone Triage tool can be customised by the user to reflect different health economies while retaining the core which is MTS.

Clinical prioritisation (whether called triage or anything else) remains a central plank of clinical risk management in all emergency care settings. This telephone iteration of a triage system which prioritises millions of patients each year provides a robust, safe, evidence-based system for managing the risk inherent in patients who are at a distance from health care providers.

Janet Marsden, Mark Newton, Jill Windle, Kevin Mackway-Jones
January 2015

CHAPTER 1

Introduction

Triage is a system of clinical risk management employed in Emergency Departments worldwide to manage patient flow safely when clinical need exceeds capacity. Systems are intended to ensure care is defined according to patient need and in a timely manner. Early Emergency Department triage was intuitive rather than methodological and was therefore neither reproducible between practitioners nor auditable.

The Manchester Triage Group was set up in November 1994 with the aim of establishing consensus amongst senior emergency physicians and emergency nurses about triage standards. It soon became apparent that the Group's aims could be set out under five headings.

1. Development of common nomenclature
2. Development of common definitions
3. Development of robust triage methodology
4. Development of training package
5. Development of audit guide for triage

Nomenclature and definitions

A review of the triage nomenclature and definitions that were in use at the time revealed considerable differences. A representative sample of these is summarised in Table 1.1.

Despite this enormous variation, it was also apparent that there were a number of common themes running through the different triage systems; these are highlighted in Table 1.2.

Emergency Triage: Telephone triage and advice, First Edition. Updated version 1.7, 2023.
Edited by Janet Marsden, Mark Newton, Jill Windle and Kevin Mackway-Jones.
© 2016 John Wiley & Sons, Ltd. Published 2016 by John Wiley & Sons, Ltd.

Table 1.1

Hospital 1		Hospital 2		Hospital 3		Hospital 4	
Red	0	A	0	Immediate	0	1	0
Amber	<15	B	<10	Urgent	5–10	2	<10
		C	<60	Semi-urgent	30–60		
Green	<120	D	<120				
Blue	<240	E	—	Delay acceptable	—	3	—
		FGHI					

Table 1.2

Priority	Maximum times (minutes)			
1	0	0	0	0
2	<15	<10	5–10	<10
3		<60	30–60	
4	120	<120		
5	<240	—	—	—

Table 1.3

Number	Name	Colour	Maximum time (minutes)
1	Immediate	Red	0
2	Very urgent	Orange	10
3	Urgent	Yellow	60
4	Standard	Green	120
5	Non-urgent	Blue	240

Once the common themes of triage had been highlighted, it became possible to quickly agree on a new common nomenclature and definition system. Each of the new categories was given a number, a colour and a name and was defined in terms of ideal maximum time to first contact with the treating clinician. At meetings between representatives of Emergency Nursing and Emergency Medicine nationally, this work informed the derivation of the United Kingdom triage scale as shown in Table 1.3.

As practice has developed over the past 20 years, five-part triage scales have been established around the world. The target times themselves are locally set, being influenced by politics as much as medicine, particularly at lower priorities, but the concept of varying clinical priority remains current.

The development of Telephone Triage

After a period where all Emergency Departments in the Manchester area were using 'Manchester Triage' and using it on the telephone to triage callers to the ED (prior to NHS Direct), it became apparent that although all Emergency Department staff were using the same language of triage, the interface with paramedic colleagues still faced a language barrier. Key collaborators within the ambulance service recognised that applications of the Manchester Triage method would be extremely useful within the ambulance service and a further group of clinicians across acute care settings and the ambulance service was set up to explore this. Telephone Triage emerged as one of the products of this collaboration and had been used successfully for both secondary triage (since 2006) and latterly primary triage (2012) of those patients accessing care by telephoning ambulance services in a number of ambulance services across the United Kingdom and internationally.

Triage methodology

In general terms, a triage method can try and provide the practitioner with the diagnosis, disposal or clinical priority. 'Manchester Triage' is designed to allocate a clinical priority. This decision was based on three major tenets. First, the aim of the triage encounter is to aid clinical management of the individual patient, and this is best achieved by accurate allocation of a clinical priority. Second, the length of the triage encounter is such that any attempts to accurately diagnose a patient are doomed to fail. Third, it is apparent that diagnosis is not accurately linked to clinical priority. The latter reflects a number of aspects of the particular patient's presentation as well as the diagnosis; for example patients with a final diagnosis of ankle sprain may present with severe or no pain and their clinical priority must reflect this. In Telephone Triage, the allocation of this clinical priority is inherently linked to a place of definitive clinical care, and in the highest priority, a mode of emergency transport to this care.

In outline, the triage method put forward in this book requires practitioners to select from a range of presentations and then to seek a limited number of signs and symptoms at each level of clinical priority. The signs and symptoms that discriminate between the clinical priorities are termed *discriminators* and they are set out in the form of flow charts for each presentation – the *presentational flow charts*. Discriminators that indicate higher levels of priority are sought first, and to a large degree, patients who are allocated to the standard clinical priority are selected by default. In this way, it reflects the effective face to face triage methodology taught by the Manchester Triage Group. The clinical priority is inherently linked to a disposal: where does the patient obtain the definitive care which they require and what is the timescale within which this must be obtained for optimum outcomes. The possible outcomes of Telephone Triage are simplified from the five categories system as there are fewer options available to the Telephone Triage practitioner.

The decisions which must be made are as follows:

- Does the patient need immediate and urgent care? (FtF Now)
- Do they need to be seen face to face by a clinician soon, but not immediately? (FtF Soon)
- Can medical or other care be delayed? (FtF Later)
- Can an 'advice only' route be followed, where the problem can be managed by giving self-care advice?

Face to face triage practitioners will note differences between the discriminators seen within face to face triage and those in the Telephone Triage method. For some discriminators used in face to face triage, it is impossible to ascertain without actually having the patient in front of the triage practitioner, whether the discriminator is fulfilled or not. Those discriminators are therefore not used in Telephone Triage. Slight changes are made to other discriminators in order for them to be more appropriate in a Telephone Triage setting.

Advice

Advice is presented on the charts at each level and is to highlight issues which can be discussed by the practitioner with the patient or caller. It is important that interim advice is given and that, if the patient is triaged to 'advice only', comprehensive advice is given and understanding is checked. The patient must know what to do should the situation change. A key premise of the advice in these charts is that it is general and may be adapted for use in specific settings. The algorithms, as in the case of the face to face algorithms, are evidence based and validated and must not be modified.

The decision making process is discussed in Chapter 2 and the triage method itself is explained in detail in Chapter 3.

Presentation priority matrix

Patients who are in the 'FtF Now' category are best served by the Emergency Ambulance Service and Emergency Departments, whatever their locations. Those requiring 'FtF Soon' or 'FtF Later' may have care delivered in a number of locations and by various providers. Thus the time to care in the 'FtF Soon' category will vary, depending upon those services available in that health economy. A mapping exercise should be undertaken locally to agree the appropriate dispositions arising from the triage decision (see Chapter 4). It is essential that the practitioner undertaking Telephone Triage is able to use up-to-date details about current local services such as dental emergency arrangements, telephone numbers of primary care facilities and the location of pharmacy provision.

Training for triage

This book and the accompanying course attempt to provide the training necessary to allow introduction of a standard triage method. It is not envisaged that reading the book and attending a course can produce instant expertise in triage. Rather this process will introduce the method and allow practitioners to develop competence at using the material available. This is the first step towards competence in using the system and must be followed up by audit and evaluation of the system in use.

Triage audit

The Triage Group spent considerable time trying to pin down 'sentinel diagnoses', that is diagnoses that could be identified retrospectively and which could be used as markers of accurate triage. For the reasons outlined above, it soon became apparent that even retrospective diagnosis could not accurately predict actual clinical priority at presentation.

Successful introduction of a robust audit method is essential to the future of any standard methodology, since reproducibility between individual practitioners and departments must be shown to exist. This is discussed in more detail in chapter 5.

Summary

Triage is a fundamental part of clinical risk management in all areas of urgent and emergency care when clinical load exceeds clinical availability. Emergency Triage promulgates a system that delivers a teachable, auditable method of assigning clinical priority in emergency settings. It is not designed to judge whether patients are appropriately in the emergency setting, but to ensure that those who need care receive it appropriately quickly. It can be used to monitor care and to signpost streams of care – these will be determined by local provision and actual availability.

CHAPTER 2

The decision making process and Telephone Triage

Introduction

Decision making is an essential and integral part of nursing and medical practice. Sound clinical judgement in relation to patient care requires both knowledge and experience. Many practitioners argue that critical decision making is only about 'common sense' and 'problem solving' and to a certain extent they are correct. It is, however, more than this and requires a high level of skill. Within the decision making process, clinicians are expected to

Interpret
Discriminate
Evaluate

the information they gather about patients and critically appraise their actions following that decision. Without a framework of reference on which to base these decisions, they will be unstructured, haphazard and potentially unsafe. The ability to make sound decisions is essential for safe and effective patient management.

Early triage systems structured the interview but gave no guidance about the action following a decision. Thus the *outcome* of the triage process was not based on a sound methodology. Triage decisions were unique to each nurse and inherently part of their own decision making process and such decisions are likely to be fundamentally flawed without a framework of reference. To overcome this problem, a framework of reference (methodology) for the process of triage and a method by which practitioners can acquire the necessary skills for its implementation are required.

Emergency Triage: Telephone triage and advice, First Edition. Updated version 1.7, 2023.
Edited by Janet Marsden, Mark Newton, Jill Windle and Kevin Mackway-Jones.
© 2016 John Wiley & Sons, Ltd. Published 2016 by John Wiley & Sons, Ltd.

The development of expertise

A relationship between experience and skill acquisition has been described in which there are five stages of development as shown below.

Novice
Advance beginner
Competent
Proficient
Expert

As practitioners develop along this continuum, they acquire skills and learn from their experiences in practice, and it is expected that their decision-making ability alters and improves. The process can be facilitated by providing a system based upon a common framework that is methodologically sound, on which decisions can be based and their effectiveness evaluated.

Decision-making strategies

A number of strategies are used in the decision-making process. They are as follows.

- Reasoning
- Pattern recognition
- Repetitive hypothesising
- Mental representation
- Intuition

Reasoning

There are essentially two types of reasoning involved in critical thinking: inductive and deductive.

Inductive reasoning is the ability to consider all possibilities and is particularly useful for the less experienced. It involves a time-consuming process of considering all patient information collected in order to reach a sound decision about the care they require.

Deductive reasoning is the simultaneous 'weeding out' of possible solutions whilst actively collecting patient information. This strategy is often unknown or unrecognised and becomes part of expert practice. It allows the practitioner to rapidly sort relevant from irrelevant information to reach a decision.

Pattern recognition

This is the strategy most commonly used by clinicians and is particularly important when making rapid decisions based on limited information that are necessary during triage. Pattern recognition is a method of piecing information together in an analytical sense. Clinicians interpret the pattern of the patient signs and symptoms by comparison with relationships and conditions from previous cases. This leads them to a decision about the patient's well-being or a potential diagnosis. The ability to use this decision making skill develops with experience and often appears to be intuition. Novice, proficient or competent practitioners may need to use conscious problem solving to reach a solution, while their more experienced colleagues can employ pattern recognition.

Repetitive hypothesising

Repetitive hypothesising is used by clinicians to test diagnostic reasoning. By gathering data to confirm or eliminate a hypothesis, a decision can be made. Depending on the level of expertise, this method can be either inductive or deductive.

Mental representation

Mental representation is a method of simplifying the situation to provide a general picture and allow focusing on relevant information. This strategy is often used when a problem is highly complex or overwhelming. The use of analogies helps the clinician visualise the situation by simplifying the problem and allowing a different perspective. Triage decisions need to be rapid and this method has limited use at this stage in the patient's pathway.

Intuition

Intuition is inextricably linked with expertise and is commonly seen as the ability of practitioners to solve problems with relatively little data. Intuition rarely involves conscious analysis and is often expressed as 'gut feeling' or 'strong hunch'. Expert practitioners view situations holistically and draw on past experience. Much of their knowledge is embedded in practice and referred to as tacit, where effective decisions are made by combining knowledge with decision-making theories and intuitive thought. Many expert clinicians are unaware of the mental processes they employ in the assessment and management of patients. Although intuition has remained unmeasurable, the value to clinical practice is acknowledged and well documented.

Decision-making during triage

Despite all the theories, decision making is quite simply a series of steps to reach a conclusion and consists of three main phases: identification of a problem, determination of the alternatives and selection of the most appropriate alternative.

An approach to making critical decisions has been described which uses the following five steps.

---

1. Identify the problem
2. Gather and analyse information related to the solution
3. Consider all the alternatives and select one for implementation
4. Implement the selected alternative
5. Monitor the implementation and evaluate outcomes

This approach incorporates a number of theories and methods. When applied to triage, the decisions are formed as follows.

Identify the problem

This is done by obtaining information from the patients or whoever is calling. Every effort should be made to talk to the patient. This phase allows the relevant presentational flow chart to be identified.

Gather and analyse information related to the solution

Once a flow chart has been identified, this phase is facilitated since discriminators can be sought at each level. The charts facilitate rapid assessment by suggesting structured questions. Pattern recognition also plays a part at this stage.

Consider all alternatives and select one for implementation

Clinicians collect significant amounts of data about the patients they deal with which is collated into their own mental database and stored in compartments for easy recall. Use of this stored information is most effective when linked to an assessment or organisational framework. The presentational flow charts provide the organisational framework to order the thought process during triage. The flow charts aid decision making by providing a structure and, importantly, support junior staff as they acquire decision-making skills.

Implement the selected alternative

There are four levels of priority (as discussed in Chapter 1) and the triage practitioner tests the discriminators against the patient's presentation and allocates priority at the highest level of positive discriminator. The priority therefore depends upon the urgency of the patient's condition and once the priority is allocated the appropriate pathway of care begins.

Monitor the implementation and evaluate outcomes

The method of triage outlined in this book ensures that the decision is predetermined if the correct process has been followed. The triage practitioner will therefore be able to identify how and why they reached the initial outcome (priority), conduct an accurate reassessment and subsequent confirmation or change in priority. Accurate, reproducible decisions ensure that the whole process can be audited.

Changing current decision-making practice

For many experienced clinicians, the introduction of a new framework for triage decisions poses some anxieties. It is difficult to unlearn individual methods of decision making which have developed over years of practice. However, this change should be viewed as a further refinement of their present system, providing for the first time a clear rationale for their decisions and an auditable system. This systematic approach will be a major contribution to the body of knowledge when used to teach junior staff, who rely so heavily on experts to inform and guide their own practice. The actual process of triage decision making presented here has been shown to be effective and adaptable to many practice settings and has value to triage practitioners irrespective of their level of experience.

CHAPTER 3
The Telephone Triage method

Introduction

The method outlined in this book is designed to allow the Telephone Triage Practitioner to rapidly assign a clinical priority to each patient. The system selects patients with the highest priority first without making any assumptions about the diagnosis. Telephone Triage prioritisation is driven by presenting signs and symptoms – it is impossible to diagnose by telephone and attempts to do so are fraught with danger.

Five-step process to triage decision making
1. Identify the problem
2. Gather and analyse information related to the solution
3. Evaluate all the alternatives and select one for implementation
4. Implement the selected alternative
5. Monitor the implementation and evaluate outcomes

Identifying the problem

Clinical practice is geared around the concept of a *presenting complaint* – that is the chief sign or symptom identified by the patient or carer. A list of presentations pertinent to Telephone triage is shown below.

Emergency Triage: Telephone triage and advice, First Edition. Updated version 1.7, 2023.
Edited by Janet Marsden, Mark Newton, Jill Windle and Kevin Mackway-Jones.
© 2016 John Wiley & Sons, Ltd. Published 2016 by John Wiley & Sons, Ltd.

Abdominal pain in adults	Irritable child
Abdominal pain in children	Limb problems
Abscesses and local infections	Limping child
Allergy	Major trauma
Apparently drunk	Medication request
Assault	Mental illness
Asthma	Neck pain
Back pain	Overdose and poisoning
Behaving strangely	Palpitations
Bites and stings	Pregnancy
Burns and scalds	PV bleeding
Chemical exposure	Rashes
Chest pain	Self-harm
Collapsed adult	Sexually acquired infection
Crying baby	Shortness of breath in adults
Dental problems	Shortness of breath in children
Diabetes	Sore throat
Diarrhoea and vomiting	Testicular pain
Ear problems	Torso injury
Eye problems	Unwell adult
Facial problems	Unwell baby
Falls	Unwell child
Fits	Unwell newborn
Foreign body	Urinary problems
GI bleed	Worried parent
Headache	Wounds
Head injury	

This list of presentational flow charts covers almost all presentations to Emergency Departments and therefore to a Telephone Triage service prior to attendance at an emergency care setting. The list, charts and contents were finalised after considerable discussion and have been refined in both this and previous editions following changes in practice, research and international consultation. The presentations fall broadly into the categories of illness, injury, children, abnormal and unusual behaviour.

The first part of the triage method requires the practitioner to select the most appropriate presentational flow chart from the list. The chart identifies discriminators which allow the clinical priority to be determined.

A key feature of the method is that the charts are consistent in their approach, as it is recognised that a number of patients' chief complaints may lead to more than one presentational flow chart. For example, a patient who feels generally unwell with a stiff neck and a headache will be given the same priority whether the practitioner uses the *Unwell Adult*, *Neck Pain* or *Headache* flow charts.

Gathering and analysing information

To a great extent, the patient's presentation elicited by the first few moments of the telephone conversation with patient or carer will dictate which presentational flow chart is selected. The Telephone Triage practitioner should ALWAYS try to speak to the patient rather than someone calling on their behalf. If the patient is unable to speak to the Telephone Triage practitioner, the practitioner should ensure that the person providing information is in visual and verbal contact with the patient. Following this selection, information must be gathered and analysed to allow the actual priority to be determined. The flow chart structures this process by showing key discriminators at each level of priority – the assessment is carried out by finding the highest level at which the answer posed by the discriminator question is positive. Discriminators are deliberately posed as questions by the triage practitioner to facilitate the process and suggestions for appropriate questions are integrated into the discriminator dictionary which begins on page 34.

Discriminators

Discriminators, as their name implies, are factors that discriminate between patients such that they allow them to be allocated to one of the five clinical priorities. They can be *General* or *Specific* and are arranged in A, B, C, D, E format. General discriminators apply to all patients irrespective of their presentation and therefore appear time and time again throughout the charts; on each occasion, the general discriminators will lead the Triage Practitioner to allocate the same clinical priority. Specific discriminators are applicable to individual presentations or to small groups of presentations and tend to relate to key features of particular conditions. Thus while *Severe pain* is a general discriminator, *Cardiac pain* and *Pleuritic pain* are specific discriminators. General discriminators appear in many more charts than specific ones. All the discriminators used are defined in the discriminator dictionary at the end of the book, and the definitions of the specific ones in use on individual charts are repeated on the accompanying chart notes for ease of reference. All discriminators are reviewed for each edition. Any changes are published on the triage web site at www.triagenet.net.

Face to face triage practitioners will note differences between the discriminators seen within face to face triage and those in the Telephone Triage method. For some discriminators used in face to face triage, it is impossible to ascertain without actually having the patient in front of the triage practitioner, whether the discriminator is fulfilled or not. Those discriminators are therefore not used in Telephone Triage. Slight changes are made to other discriminators in order for them to be more appropriate in a Telephone Triage setting.

General discriminators are a recurring feature of the charts, and a proper understanding of them is essential to an understanding of the triage method. Six general discriminators are discussed further here – these are shown in the box.

1. Life threat
2. Haemorrhage
3. Conscious level
4. Temperature
5. Pain
6. Acuteness

Life threat

Life threat is perhaps the most obvious general discriminator of all. Broadly speaking this recognises that any cessation or threat to the vital (ABC) functions places the patient in priority 1 (Red – FtF Now).

Patients who are unable to maintain their own airway for any length of time have an insecure airway. Additionally, patients with stridor have significant airway threat – this may be an inspiratory or expiratory noise, or both. Stridor is heard best on breathing with the mouth open. Inadequacy of breathing includes absence (defined as no respiration or respiratory effort as assessed by looking, listening and feeling for 10 seconds) and includes patients who are failing to breathe well enough to maintain adequate oxygenation. There may be an increased work of breathing, signs of inadequate breathing or exhaustion.

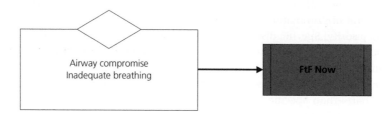

Haemorrhage

Haemorrhage is a feature of many presentations – particularly, but not exclusively, those involving trauma. The haemorrhage discriminators in Telephone Triage are uncontrolled major and uncontrolled minor. The use of the success of attempts to control haemorrhage is deliberate as, in general, continuing bleeding has a higher clinical priority. While of course in practice it can be difficult to decide which category a particular haemorrhage falls into, the definitions of the discriminators are designed to help the practitioner to do this. A haemorrhage that is not rapidly controlled by the application of sustained direct pressure, and in which blood continues to flow heavily or soak through large dressings quickly, is described as an uncontrollable major haemorrhage. A haemorrhage in which blood continues to flow slightly or ooze is described as uncontrollable minor haemorrhage.

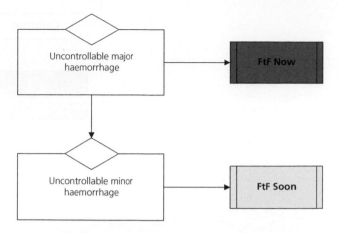

Conscious level

Conscious level is considered differently for adults and children. In adults only currently fitting patients and those with an altered conscious level are always categorised as priority 1 (Red – FtF Now), while all unresponsive children are placed in this clinical priority. All patients with a history of unconsciousness should be allocated to priority 2 (Yellow – FtF Soon).

The fact that all patients with alterations in conscious level are allocated to the 'FtF Now' priority may be at odds with current practice; this is especially so with regard to the clinical priority given to patients who are intoxicated or under the influence of drugs.

Two points need to be made about this. First, the aetiology of alterations in level of consciousness is largely irrelevant in determining the risk to the patient – an altered conscious level due to drugs or alcohol is clinically as important as altered conscious level due to other causes. Second, most drunk patients do not have an altered level of consciousness. Specific points about the allocation of clinical priority to patients who are apparently drunk are dealt with in the presentational flow chart of that name.

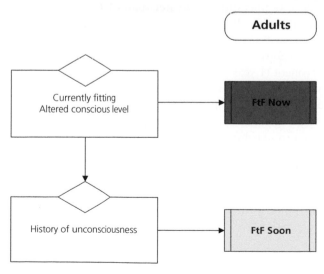

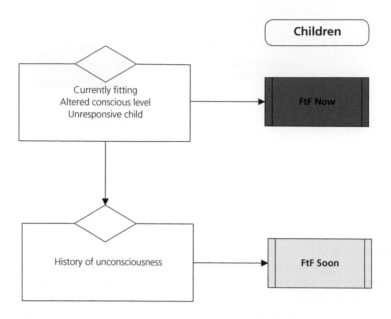

Temperature

Temperature is used as a general discriminator. Although accurate measurement of temperature may be difficult to achieve in practice, many parents employ various types of temperature measuring device to assess temperature in children.

Clinical impression of skin temperature is important and is crucial where immediate assessment of core temperature is not possible. This cannot be ascertained by telephone but only by **very** careful questioning and should be used with caution where an **actual** temperature is not available. Other signs of pyrexia such as rigors and feeling very cold should be taken into account when assessing temperature by telephone.

If the skin is very hot, then the patient is clinically said to be very hot – this corresponds to a temperature of greater than 41°C; similarly if the skin is hot, then the patient is clinically said to be hot and this corresponds to a temperature of greater than 38.5°C. A patient with warm skin fulfils the discriminator of warmth and this goes with a temperature of less than 38.5°C.

A very hot patient (1 year and above) will always be categorised as priority 1 (Red – FtF Now), whilst a hot patient will be categorised as priority 2 (Yellow – FtF Soon). Patients who are cold will be allocated to priority 1 (Red – FtF Now). The hot baby (from birth to 12 months) will always be categorised as priority 1 (Red – FtF Now) and the warm newborn (a baby of 28 days old or less) as priority 2 (Yellow – FtF Soon).

	Very Hot 41°C or more	Hot 38.5°C or more	Warm 37.5°C or more
Newborn (up to 28 days)			
Baby (child of 12 months or less)			
Child over 12 months			
Adult			

Pain

From the patients' perspective, pain is a major factor in determining priority. The use of pain as a general discriminator throughout the presentational flow charts recognises this fact and implies that every Telephone Triage assessment should include an assessment of pain. Because accurate assessment of pain is almost impossible in Telephone Triage, there are only two categories of pain recordable in this system. In general terms, the discriminator severe pain is intended to imply pain that is unbearable, often described as the worst ever. Any patient with a lesser degree of pain is recorded as 'unresolved pain' which is defined as pain which has not resolved despite waiting an appropriate time or being given appropriate analgesia. This patient should, if no other discriminators suggest a higher categorisation, be allocated priority 3 (Green – FtF Later) and not be allocated to an 'advice only' category.

The general pain discriminator describes the intensity or severity of pain only. Other characteristics of pain, such as site, radiation and periodicity, may feature as specific discriminators in particular presentational flow charts.

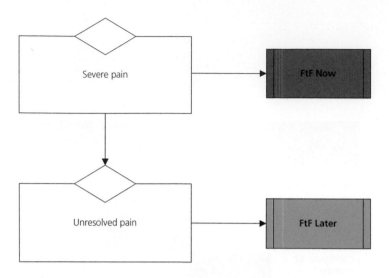

Acuteness

Within the triage method, certain conventions have been used to help with consistency. The term 'abrupt' is used to indicate onset within seconds or minutes and 'acute' indicates a time period within 24 hours. Recent symptoms and signs are those that have appeared within the past 7 days.

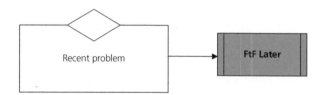

Evaluating alternatives and selecting one

Selection of the most appropriate flow chart presents a number of general and specific discriminators which can then be tested against the patient. The skill in implementing the triage method lies in the application of this testing. Practitioners must decide whether the criteria for the presence of each discriminator is fulfilled and must decide which discriminator is the most applicable at the highest clinical priority. For example, for the adult who presents with abdominal pain and complains of persistent vomiting and is hot (both priority 2 – FtF Soon), the most appropriate discriminator is *persistent vomiting* as this provides more significant information about this patient.

Implementing the selected alternative

This step is essentially a procedural one. The inevitable outcome of the information gathering, analysis and evaluation leads to allocation of one of the clinical priorities shown in the box.

Number	Name	Colour
1	FtF Now	Red
2	FtF Soon	Yellow
3	FtF Later	Green
4	Advice only	Blue

Documentation

Implementation involves recording the allocated priority and showing the decision making that led to it. The triage method outlined here allows documentation to be simple and precise. The minimum required is a record of which presentational flow chart is being used, which discriminator defines the category and which category has been selected. Thus, for instance, the triage record of a patient with chest pain might be as shown in the box.

Chest pain Pleuritic pain FtF Soon (yellow)

This simple approach to documentation allows for simple audit but it is recognised that computer decision support software is widely used and will dictate the way the triage event is recorded.

Patient assessment

The purist view of the triage event is a rapid and focussed encounter in which information is gathered and applied to assign a priority. This type of assessment is a skill in itself and carries a higher degree of risk when undertaken without the ability to actually see the patient and when, on many occasions, the person making the telephone call is not actually the patient.

The following framework can be used to teach the process to Telephone Triage practitioners, ensuring decisions are based on relevant and appropriate patient data.

It is important that the assessment of a patient is systematic and all elements of that assessment are pieced together to give a complete picture of the patient's problem. For this reason, the Telephone Triage practitioner should have sufficient experience of urgent/emergency care and the interpersonal skills to communicate effectively with patients and their families and carers.

The approach to this assessment should take the following format (Table 3.1):

By following this systematic process, facilitated by the triage methodology, patient assessment can be performed rapidly and confidently to reach an appropriate clinical priority in order to guide decision making.

Table 3.1

Assessment component	Triage activity
Greeting the patient/caller	Listen to voice
	Ascertain whether patient or other and if possible, ask to speak to the patient
Patient history	Ask the patient what the problem is
	This is a short, concise, subjective history and tells you about the patient's injury/illness/health-related problem
Presenting complaint	Patients' presenting complaint can be established from the subjective history they provide
	This leads the triage practitioner to choose the most appropriate presentation flow chart
Focused questions (interview)	This is where the triage practitioners' knowledge and skills are most evident. Application of anatomical knowledge, pattern recognition of presenting complaints and the ability to react effectively to life-threatening situations are all the domain of the triage practitioner
	Focused questions can be used to obtain more detail if required, for example mechanism of injury, duration of the problem and current medications. *The format of these questions will be directed by the discriminators in the chosen presentation flow chart*
Physical examination and assessment of physical parameters	Physical examination and assessment of physical parameters is possible during face to face triage but less so on the end of a telephone, but some questions such as the following could be asked:
	What things sound like – *do they make a gurgling sound when they breathe*?
	What things look like – *does the limb look a different colour when you compare it to the other side*?
	What things feel like – *do they feel hot or cold to the touch*?
	What effect the problem is having – *is your vision blurred or strange*?
Pain assessment	Pain assessment in Telephone Triage is difficult so pain has been revised to:
	• Severe pain (FtF now)
	• Unresolved pain (pain which has not resolved despite the use of appropriate analgesia) in the absence of any other discriminator (FtF later)

Table 3.1 (*Continued*)

Assessment component	Triage activity
	This can only be assessed by asking the patient directly and perhaps comparing the pain being experienced with pain experienced in the past.
Priority/plan of care	Priority assigned using the highest discriminator applicable to the patient
	Decisions made about where the patient will be seen, what transport decisions have been made
	Relevant advice given
	What to do if things get worse
Documentation	The recording of this information should be to an agreed format and again clear, concise and relevant to the presenting complaint
	Include a record of any: • Allergies • Current medications • Relevant past medical history • Relevant social issues

Checking for understanding

It is absolutely crucial that the patient, or the person calling on behalf of the patient, understands the information and advice being given by the Telephone Triage practitioner, and checking for understanding should be a continual part of the process.

Interim advice

As the patient is remote from the triage practitioner, interim advice maybe necessary in order to promote recovery or prevent deterioration in the condition of the patient before face to face assessment. For example, if the triage practitioner obtains information that the patient is not breathing effectively or has airway compromise, then life-saving basic life support advice must be given to the caller so that resuscitation can be attempted until help arrives. Similarly, if a child is unwell and is triaged to 'medicine later' it may be appropriate to give the carer advice on simple measures to alleviate symptoms such as fever and diarrhoea. Each chart shows interim advice which can be added to depending on the local requirement.

Advice only

In the advice only category, tailored advice should be given to the patient and checked for understanding.

The advice which should be provided to the patient by the Telephone Triage practitioner (as appropriate) for the chart 'Abdominal Pain in Adults' is summarized below.

FtF Now	FtF Soon	FtF Later	Advice only
Provide life support advice if required	Take available analgesia for pain control	Maintain hydration with clear fluids or oral rehydration therapy	Maintain fluid intake – plenty of clear fluids/consider oral rehydration therapy
Take available analgesia for pain control	Call back if symptoms worsen or concerned	Take available analgesia for pain control	Paracetamol qds for pain and temperature control
Keep sample of vomit/stool if possible	Keep sample of stool if possible	Call back if symptoms worsen or concerned	Rest
			Refer to GP if symptoms persist
			Call back if symptoms worsen or concerned

A key premise of the advice in these charts is that it is general and may be adapted for use in specific settings. The algorithms, as in the case of the face to face algorithms, are evidence based and validated and must not be altered.

Monitoring and evaluating

Understanding should be checked by questioning and the patient asked if they have any questions for the practitioner, before the Telephone Triage episode is complete.

It is important that callers are given information about what to do if things change and the evaluation, particularly of 'advice only' decisions, may be undertaken by patient call back and continuous audit.

CHAPTER 4
The presentation priority matrix

The Manchester Triage System was designed to be a robust, auditable clinical risk management tool that identified the clinical priority of individual patients. As has been alluded to earlier in this book, the process itself and the outcome of the process can be useful beyond prioritisation.

Presentation-priority matrix mapping

As the idea of the inappropriate patient becomes replaced by the concepts of inappropriate care delivery and patient choice, multiple entry gates to emergency care and the 'emergency care village' become realities. Clinicians must be equipped with tools that enable them to decide safely and effectively where patients might be best managed.

In Telephone Triage, it is crucial that the outcome of the prioritisation process informs decisions about the most appropriate disposition of the patient. In particular, the combination of the presentational chart used and the priority allocated (the presentation-priority matrix) should be matched to particular types of provision of emergency care so that every patient with a particular outcome is dealt with in an appropriate, effective and consistent way. This outcome will be different depending on the locality, time of day and services available at that time. Thus a patient presenting, by telephone, with a limb problem and allocated to the 'Face-to-Face (FtF) Soon' priority could be seen in a minor injury unit, in the Emergency Department (ED) or in primary care, while a patient with chest pain allocated to the 'FtF Now' will always have an emergency ambulance dispatched and be taken to an Emergency Department. The MTS consists of 53 presentations and up to 3 priorities – making a total of 155 presentation-priority combinations.

Emergency Triage: Telephone triage and advice, First Edition. Updated version 1.7, 2023.
Edited by Janet Marsden, Mark Newton, Jill Windle and Kevin Mackway-Jones.
© 2016 John Wiley & Sons, Ltd. Published 2016 by John Wiley & Sons, Ltd.

A mapping exercise should be undertaken with all providers of care to consider appropriate disposition of all of these and a consensus reached with clinicians in all areas so that all patients reach appropriate face to face assessment and care.

Explanation of the process

When making decisions as to the most appropriate disposition for patients, it is important to identify a range of stakeholders who will work to develop the matrix finally reaching a consensus decision. Where patients will be directed across a range of services, it is useful to engage different providers and different professionals, job roles to give a balanced view of how patients will be directed.

Completing the PPM

- Establish the list of dispositions to which patients can be directed (see examples below).
- Provide each stakeholder with a blank matrix and a copy of Emergency Triage: Telephone Triage and Advice; this is strictly an open book exercise to ensure each stakeholder bases their decisions on the same methodology the Telephone Triage practitioners will be using.
- The stakeholders will individually use a reductionist approach (start at priority 1 – FtF Now – and work along the priorities to priority 4 – Advice Only) to consider for each of the presentation charts which disposition is appropriate for the patient in a particular priority, for example

  Unwell Adult – Priority 1 – FtF Now – inadequate breathing = Despatch of Emergency Ambulance

  Dental problems – Priority 3 – FtF Later – unresolved pain = Primary Care or Dental Service

- All completed matrices collated, where consensus not reached further iteration required until a clear map of agreed dispositions is produced.
- This process can and should be repeated at intervals to ensure any change in services is represented in the matrix.

The dispositions

A large ambulance service disposition matrix using presentation and priority is shown here. The dispositions available will be subject to local emergency care provision. For example, the lack of an emergency eye unit, or the fact that one exists but is not open 24 hours a day, will change where patients with eye problems are managed. It may, however, also stimulate debate with the local ophthalmic service in order to provide a more appropriate service for these patients. The dispositions shown below, assume a complete range of emergency care provision. The Telephone Triage practitioner will need to exercise judgement as to which is the most appropriate. This decision will be influenced by the availability of the services, the current pressures on them, the triage discriminator and perhaps the patient's choice or their ability to travel to a service.

Experience has shown that triage must be accurate (as assessed by audit) if it is to be used to drive disposition.

Times to 'face to face'

The times associated with each of these outcomes will be driven by a number of factors including local emergency provision as well as locally and nationally driven priorities and targets. What is clear is that 'FtF Now' will always require urgent care as quickly as is possible in the prevailing circumstances and it may be agreed locally that the Telephone Triage professional remains in contact with the patient or the caller until appropriate help arrives.

Key/definitions for this PPM:

- ED – Emergency Department or Urgent Care Centre (condition dependent)
- EDC – Emergency Dental Centre and/or Own Transport
- EEC – Emergency Eye Centre and/or Own Transport
- MAT – Maternity Services (e.g. labour ward, early pregnancy unit)
- MIU – Minor Injuries Unit or Walk-In Centre and/or Own Transport
- PA – Psychiatric Assessment
- PC – Primary Care Emergency Centre (e.g. GP-led walk-in facility, GP Surgery) and/or Own Transport
- SC – Self Care Advice and/or PC referral greater than 4 hours
- SHC – Sexual Health Clinic or G.U.M Service and/or Own Transport

Presentation	'FtF Now' outcome	'FtF Soon' outcome	'FtF Later' outcome
Abdominal pain (adult)	ED	Consider PC	PC
Abdominal pain (child)	ED	ED	PC
Abscesses and local infections	ED	Consider PC	PC
Allergy	ED	PC	SC
Apparently drunk			
Assault	ED	Consider MIU	PC or MIU
Asthma	ED	Consider PC	PC
Back pain	ED	ED	PC or MIU
Behaving strangely	ED	ED	Consider PA or PC
Bites and stings	ED	Consider PC	PC or SC
Burns and scalds	ED	ED	PC or SC
Chemical exposure			
Chest pain	ED	Consider PC	PC
Collapsed adult	ED	ED	PC
Crying baby	ED	ED	PC
Dental problems	ED	EDC	EDC
Diabetes	ED	ED	PC
Diarrhoea and vomiting	ED	Consider PC	SC

Presentation	'FtF Now' outcome	'FtF Soon' outcome	'FtF Later' outcome
Ear problems	ED	ED	PC
Eye problems	ED	EEC	PC
Facial problems	ED	ED	PC or MIU
Falls	ED	ED	PC or MIU
Fits	ED	ED	Consider SC
Foreign body	ED	Consider PC or MIU	PC or MIU
GI bleed	ED	Consider PC	PC
Headache	ED	ED	PC
Head injury	ED	ED	Consider PC
Irritable child	ED	ED	PC
Limb problems	ED	ED	PC or MIU
Limping child	ED	ED	PC
Major Trauma			
Medication request	N/A	PC	PC
Mental illness	ED	ED or consider PA	ED or consider PA
Neck pain	ED	ED	PC or MIU
Overdose and poisoning	ED	ED	Consider PA
Palpitations	ED	ED	Consider PC
Pregnancy	ED or MAT	ED or MAT	PC or MAT
PV bleeding	ED or MAT	ED or MAT	PC
Rashes	ED	ED	PC or SC
Self-harm	ED	ED or PA	N/A
Sexually acquired infection	ED	Consider PC	PC or SHC
Shortness of breath (adult)	ED	Consider PC	PC
Shortness of breath (child)	ED	ED	PC
Sore throat	ED	PC	SC
Testicular pain	ED	ED	PC or SHC
Torso injury	ED	Consider PC	PC or MIU
Unwell adult	ED	Consider PC	PC
Unwell baby			
Unwell child	ED	ED	PC
Unwell newborn			
Urinary problems	ED	Consider PC	PC
Worried Parent	ED	ED	PC
Wounds	ED	ED or MIU	PC or MIU

Example of a priority matrix used by an ambulance service taking into account local services and transport options.

CHAPTER 5

Ensuring safety in Telephone Triage

Introduction

Telephone Triage carries more risk than face to face triage because the practitioner has no clues other than what they are able to ascertain by conversation with the person at the other end of the telephone, who may not be the patient. It is absolutely crucial then that all staff undertaking Telephone Triage are appropriately trained, assessed to ensure competence and that continuous audit is undertaken to ensure that both individual practitioners and the service as a whole remain safe and effective. Standard Operating Procedures should be formulated within the organisation in which Telephone Triage takes place to ensure that all processes are in place and approved before Telephone Triage begins to be used. When the Manchester Triage Group set out its aims at its very first meeting in November 1994, it clearly identified the need for a robust audit methodology. The reasons for this were very simple that the MTS was designed to reduce unwarranted variations in the triage process and this reduction could only be ensured by audit. Audit, in this context at least, is a quality management procedure; since triage is a fundamental cornerstone of clinical risk management, failure to ensure the quality of triage may have serious consequences.

Fortunately, the Manchester Triage methodology in its telephone as well as its face to face iteration is eminently auditable. The presentation – discriminator – priority progression (the process) by which individual triage practitioners arrive at their conclusions is very easy for an auditor to note and easily assessable for accuracy by a trained assessor. The nature of Telephone Triage is often driven by the need to effectively prioritise resources. Clinicians may be disproportionately focused on avoiding the use of emergency (scarce) resources rather than clinical quality.

Emergency Triage: Telephone triage and advice, First Edition. Updated version 1.7, 2023.
Edited by Janet Marsden, Mark Newton, Jill Windle and Kevin Mackway-Jones.
© 2016 John Wiley & Sons, Ltd. Published 2016 by John Wiley & Sons, Ltd.

Audit should therefore be weighted towards quality measures to ensure patient safety and observe principles of good clinical governance.

Appropriate training

Practitioners undertaking Telephone Triage must be experienced in the face to face aspects of their profession. Like face to face triage described within the Manchester Triage System, Telephone Triage is an expert system, designed for use by experienced practitioners rather than a simple algorithm designed for non-professional personnel. It requires very specific clinical information and the practitioners must be very skilled in telephone questioning techniques in order to ascertain the information required to make appropriate decisions and to ensure that the caller understands any instructions given.

Supervision by an experienced practitioner should be available at all times during the training process and appropriate supervision should be available even after the practitioner has been deemed competent to ensure that practitioners have clinical advice should they have difficulty with a particular call.

Competence assessment

All practitioners must be assessed for theoretical competence as well as for practical competence and should have a period of mentoring by an experienced practitioner before they are able to take calls alone.

Audit method

At a basic level, the accuracy of individual triage practitioners underpins the whole quality agenda. Thus, the most robust triage audit continuously assesses the practitioners for accuracy (and is linked by reflective practice and, if necessary, additional training to improve performance). The method outlined below is an audit of individual practitioner triage activity and is designed to audit the quality of decision making against the MTS standard, along with standards of record keeping and documentation.

- All triage practitioners are identified
- All episodes of triage are identified
- Episodes are all assigned to individual practitioners
- Two percent of episodes per practitioner (minimum of 10 episodes) are randomly selected
- Episodes are assessed by a senior trained triage practitioner
- The completeness of episodes is expressed as a simple proportion
- The accuracy of episodes is expressed as a simple proportion
- The number of incomplete episodes is fed back to the practitioner
- The overall accuracy is fed back to the practitioner
- Any causes of inaccurate triage are fed back to the practitioner

Table 5.1

Criteria	Yes	No	Comments
Correct use of presentational flow chart			
Specific discriminators			*(Record as seen on triage record)*
Correct disposition category			
Disposition communicated to patient			
Correct advice given			

To ensure consistency of audit, 10% of episodes assessed are performed independently by a second senior practitioner. Any differences are moderated by discussion. Continuous audit can be time-consuming but is an excellent means of assessing standards of triage activity and decision making (Table 5.1).

As can be seen from this, two measures of the triage process are obtained: completeness and accuracy. These are defined in the following.

Completeness

An episode is complete if all the steps necessary to reach the conclusion have been undertaken. As the method is reductive (that is it assumes everybody is priority 1 and works down from there), this requires that the practitioner excludes all the discriminators in any higher priority. Thus, if pain appears as a discriminator in the chart selected, then the episode would be incomplete if no result was recorded. Advice must be given to the patient about what disposition has been chosen and how it will be operationalised (an ambulance has been despatched, make your way to your local walk-in centre, make an appointment to see your doctor in the morning, etc.) and the record is not complete unless this has been communicated to the patient or caller and advice given in the meantime.

Accuracy

An episode is recorded as accurate if both presentation and discriminator selected are appropriate and if correct advice has been given to the patient. It is important to realise that there may be appropriate alternatives (indeed the system is designed to ensure that this can occur); thus audit should be carried out by a practitioner with sufficient experience to make this judgement.

Targets

- 0% episodes incomplete
- 95% accuracy
- 95% agreement between assessors

Triage in practice

The triage audit will have a number of additional effects on the triage process. It is not possible to carry out the audit without accurate triage notes, call recordings, or indeed, both; any deficiencies in record making will be highlighted. Feedback on a regular basis will improve these assessments. Experience has shown that this is an early 'win' from audit.

Peer review

Audit is a more powerful tool if it is undertaken by peers as well as by managers. A peer audit allows open discussion and reflective learning to take place and must be an integral part of triage audit.

System review

In Telephone Triage, it is also important to find out what happened to the patient after the practitioner has finished the Telephone Triage episode so follow-up of patients must take place.

We suggest the following in the initial phases of adoption of a Telephone Triage system:
- 10% of patients who were triaged to 'FtF Now' should be followed up, the face to face priority matched with the Telephone Triage priority
- 10% of 'FtF Soon' and 'FtF Later' followed up, matching the telephone priority against face to face triage, or a simulation of a face to face priority based on the presenting complaint
- 100% of 'Advice Only' patient should be followed up with a telephone call in a few days to ensure that the decision made was correct.

This should be part of the implementation process. Once Telephone Triage is established successfully, the degree of audit can be determined locally. The suggested percentages for individual audit may also prove onerous if Telephone Triage is undertaken for the whole of a health economy and a decision may be made locally to change these. It must be remembered though that this follow-up of Telephone Triage is vitally important to ensure that the decision, in particular, to categorise patients as 'Advice only' is safe.

Presentational Flow Chart Index

Emergency Triage: Telephone triage and advice, First Edition. Updated version 1.7, 2023.
Edited by Janet Marsden, Mark Newton, Jill Windle and Kevin Mackway-Jones.
© 2016 John Wiley & Sons, Ltd. Published 2016 by John Wiley & Sons, Ltd.

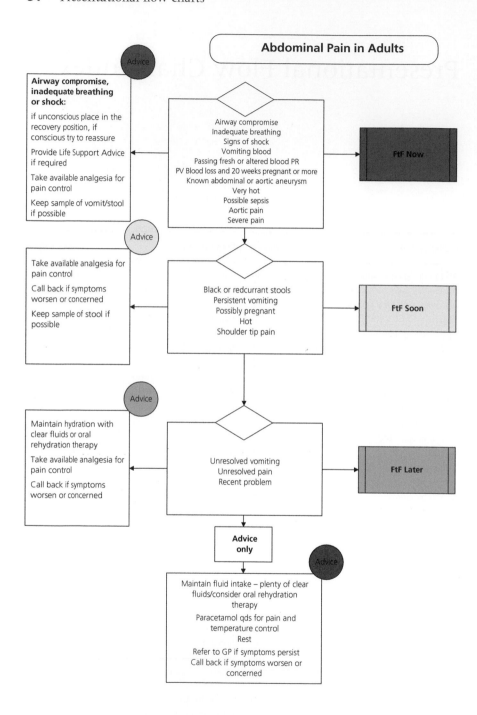

Abdominal Pain in Adults

Advice

Airway compromise, inadequate breathing or shock:

if unconscious place in the recovery position, if conscious try to reassure

Provide Life Support Advice if required

Take available analgesia for pain control

Keep sample of vomit/stool if possible

Airway compromise
Inadequate breathing
Signs of shock
Vomiting blood
Passing fresh or altered blood PR
PV Blood loss and 20 weeks pregnant or more
Known abdominal or aortic aneurysm
Very hot
Possible sepsis
Aortic pain
Severe pain

FtF Now

Advice

Take available analgesia for pain control

Call back if symptoms worsen or concerned

Keep sample of stool if possible

Black or redcurrant stools
Persistent vomiting
Possibly pregnant
Hot
Shoulder tip pain

FtF Soon

Advice

Maintain hydration with clear fluids or oral rehydration therapy

Take available analgesia for pain control

Call back if symptoms worsen or concerned

Unresolved vomiting
Unresolved pain
Recent problem

FtF Later

Advice only

Advice

Maintain fluid intake – plenty of clear fluids/consider oral rehydration therapy

Paracetamol qds for pain and temperature control

Rest

Refer to GP if symptoms persist
Call back if symptoms worsen or concerned

Abdominal pain in adults

See also	Chart notes
Diarrhoea and vomiting GI bleeding Pregnancy	This is a presentation-defined flow diagram. Abdominal pain is a common cause of presentation. A number of general discriminators are used including *Life Threat* and *Pain*. Specific discriminators are included in the 'face to face Now' and 'face to face Soon' categories to ensure that the more severe pathologies are appropriately triaged. In particular, discriminators are included to ensure that patients with moderate and severe GI bleeding and those with signs of retroperitoneal or diaphragmatic irritation are given sufficiently high categorisation

Specific discriminators	Explanation
Vomiting blood	Vomited blood may be fresh (bright or dark red) or coffee ground in appearance
Passing fresh or altered blood PR	In active massive GI bleeding, dark red blood will be passed PR. As GI transit time increases, this becomes darker, eventually becoming melaena
PV blood loss and 20 weeks pregnant or more	Any loss of blood per vaginum in a woman is known to be beyond the 20th week of pregnancy
Known abdominal or aortic aneurysm	Self (or caller) reported to have abdominal or aortic aneurysm
Possible sepsis	Suspected sepsis in patients who present with altered mental state, low blood pressure (Systolic less than 100) or raised respiratory rate (rate more than 22). In children, age specific physiological tools should be used to determine if possibly septic
Aortic pain	The onset of symptoms is sudden and the leading symptom is severe abdominal or chest pain. The pain may be described as sharp, stabbing or ripping in character. Classically aortic chest pain is felt around the sternum and then radiates to the shoulder blades, aortic abdominal pain is felt in the centre of the abdomen and radiates to the back. The pain may get better or even vanish and then recur elsewhere. Over time, pain may also be felt in the arms, neck, lower jaw, stomach or hips
Black or redcurrant stools	Any blackness fulfils the criteria of black stool while a dark red stool, classically seen in intussusceptions, is redcurrant stool
Persistent vomiting	Vomiting that is continuous or that occurs without any respite between episodes
Possibly pregnant	Any woman whose normal menstruation has failed to occur is possibly pregnant. Furthermore, any woman of childbearing age who has unprotected sex should be considered to be potentially pregnant
Shoulder tip pain	Pain felt in the tip of the shoulder. This often indicates diaphragmatic irritation
Unresolved vomiting	Vomiting which has not resolved, despite any appropriate actions

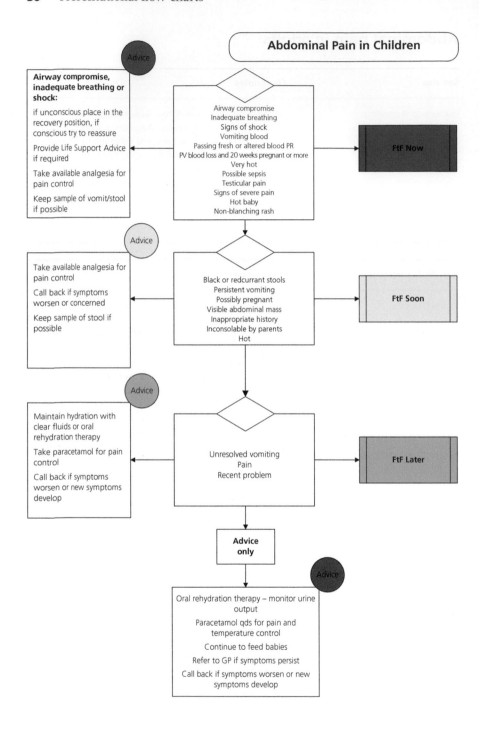

Abdominal Pain in Children

Advice

Airway compromise, inadequate breathing or shock:

if unconscious place in the recovery position, if conscious try to reassure

Provide Life Support Advice if required

Take available analgesia for pain control

Keep sample of vomit/stool if possible

Airway compromise
Inadequate breathing
Signs of shock
Vomiting blood
Passing fresh or altered blood PR
PV blood loss and 20 weeks pregnant or more
Very hot
Possible sepsis
Testicular pain
Signs of severe pain
Hot baby
Non-blanching rash

FtF Now

Advice

Take available analgesia for pain control

Call back if symptoms worsen or concerned

Keep sample of stool if possible

Black or redcurrant stools
Persistent vomiting
Possibly pregnant
Visible abdominal mass
Inappropriate history
Inconsolable by parents
Hot

FtF Soon

Advice

Maintain hydration with clear fluids or oral rehydration therapy

Take paracetamol for pain control

Call back if symptoms worsen or new symptoms develop

Unresolved vomiting
Pain
Recent problem

FtF Later

**Advice
only**

Advice

Oral rehydration therapy – monitor urine output

Paracetamol qds for pain and temperature control

Continue to feed babies

Refer to GP if symptoms persist

Call back if symptoms worsen or new symptoms develop

Abdominal pain in children

See also	Chart notes
Diarrhoea and vomiting	This is a presentation-defined flow diagram. Children who present with abdominal pain may have a range of pathologies and this chart has been designed to allow them to be accurately prioritised. A number of general discriminators are used including *Life Threat* and *Pain*. Specific discriminators are included to ensure the children who are actively bleeding, and those who have the signs or symptoms of more severe pathologies such as intussusception are given immediate care. If the patient is under 28 days, the Unwell newborn chart should be used.

Specific discriminators	Explanation
Vomiting blood	Vomited blood may be fresh (bright or dark red) or coffee ground in appearance
Passing fresh or altered blood PR	In active massive GI bleeding, dark red blood will be passed PR. As GI transit time increases, this becomes darker, eventually becoming melaena
PV blood loss and 20 weeks pregnant or more	Any loss of blood per vaginum in a woman known to be beyond the 20th week of pregnancy
Possible sepsis	Suspected sepsis in patients who present with altered mental state, low blood pressure (Systolic less than 100) or raised respiratory rate (rate more than 22). In children, age specific physiological tools should be used to determine if possibly septic
Testicular pain	Pain in the testicles
Non-blanching rash	A rash that does not blanch (go white) when pressure is applied to it. Often tested using a glass tumbler to apply pressure as any colour change can be observed through the bottom of the tumbler
Black or redcurrant stools	Any blackness fulfils the criteria of black stool while a dark red stool, classically seen in intussusceptions, is redcurrant stool
Persistent vomiting	Vomiting that is continuous or that occurs without any respite between episodes
Possibly pregnant	Any woman whose normal menstruation has failed to occur is possibly pregnant. Furthermore, any woman of childbearing age who has unprotected sex should be considered to be potentially pregnant
Visible abdominal mass	A mass in the abdomen that is visible to the naked eye
Inappropriate history	When the history (story) given does not explain the physical findings, it is termed inappropriate. This is important as it is a marker of safeguarding concerns in both adults and children
Inconsolable by parents	Children whose crying or distress does not respond to attempts by their parents to comfort them fulfil this criterion
Unresolved vomiting	Vomiting which has not resolved, despite any appropriate actions

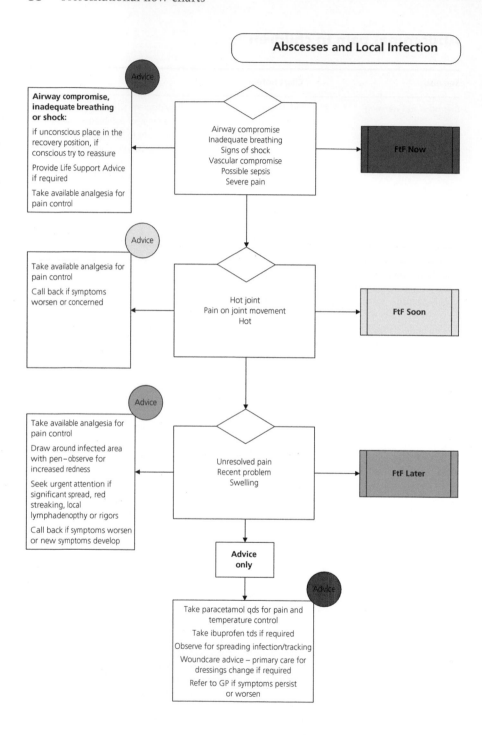

Abscesses and Local Infection

Airway compromise, inadequate breathing or shock:

if unconscious place in the recovery position, if conscious try to reassure

Provide Life Support Advice if required

Take available analgesia for pain control

Advice

Airway compromise
Inadequate breathing
Signs of shock
Vascular compromise
Possible sepsis
Severe pain

FtF Now

Take available analgesia for pain control

Call back if symptoms worsen or concerned

Advice

Hot joint
Pain on joint movement
Hot

FtF Soon

Take available analgesia for pain control

Draw around infected area with pen – observe for increased redness

Seek urgent attention if significant spread, red streaking, local lymphadenopthy or rigors

Call back if symptoms worsen or new symptoms develop

Advice

Unresolved pain
Recent problem
Swelling

FtF Later

Advice only

Advice

Take paracetamol qds for pain and temperature control

Take ibuprofen tds if required

Observe for spreading infection/tracking

Woundcare advice – primary care for dressings change if required

Refer to GP if symptoms persist or worsen

Abscesses and local infections

See also	Chart notes
Bites and stings	This is a presentation-defined flow diagram designed to allow prioritisation of patients who present with a variety of local infections and abscesses. Underlying conditions may vary from life-threatening orbital cellulitis to acneiform spots. A number of general discriminators are used including *Life Threat*, *Pain* and *Temperature*. Specific discriminators have been included to allow identification of more urgent conditions such as gas gangrene and septic arthritis

Specific discriminators	Explanation
Vascular compromise	There will be a combination of pallor, coldness, altered sensation and pain with or without absent pulses distal to the injury
Possible sepsis	Suspected sepsis in patients who present with altered mental state, low blood pressure (Systolic less than 100) or raised respiratory rate (rate more than 22). In children, age specific physiological tools should be used to determine if possibly septic
Hot joint	Any warmth around a joint fulfils this criterion; often accompanied by redness
Pain on joint movement	This can be pain on either active (patient) movement or passive (examiner) movement

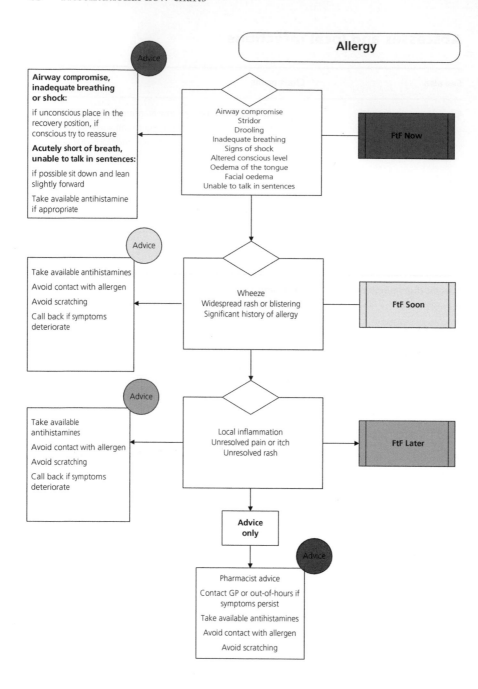

Allergy

Advice

Airway compromise, inadequate breathing or shock:

if unconscious place in the recovery position, if conscious try to reassure

Acutely short of breath, unable to talk in sentences:

if possible sit down and lean slightly forward

Take available antihistamine if appropriate

Airway compromise
Stridor
Drooling
Inadequate breathing
Signs of shock
Altered conscious level
Oedema of the tongue
Facial oedema
Unable to talk in sentences

FtF Now

Advice

Take available antihistamines

Avoid contact with allergen

Avoid scratching

Call back if symptoms deteriorate

Wheeze
Widespread rash or blistering
Significant history of allergy

FtF Soon

Advice

Take available antihistamines

Avoid contact with allergen

Avoid scratching

Call back if symptoms deteriorate

Local inflammation
Unresolved pain or itch
Unresolved rash

FtF Later

Advice only

Advice

Pharmacist advice

Contact GP or out-of-hours if symptoms persist

Take available antihistamines

Avoid contact with allergen

Avoid scratching

Allergy

See also	Chart notes
Asthma Bites and stings Collapsed adult Unwell adult	This is a presentation-defined flow diagram designed to allow prioritisation of patients with symptoms and signs that may indicate allergy. Patients with allergic reactions range from those with life-threatening anaphylaxis to those with an itchy insect bite. A number of general discriminators are used including *Life Threat*, *Conscious Level* and *Pain*. Specific discriminators have been included to allow prioritization of the most urgent conditions

Specific discriminators	Explanation
Stridor	This may be an inspiratory or expiratory noise or both. Stridor is best heard on breathing with the mouth open
Drooling	Saliva running from the mouth as a result of being unable to swallow
Oedema of the tongue	Swelling of the tongue of any degree
Facial oedema	Diffuse swelling around the face usually involving the lips
Unable to talk in sentences	Patients who are so breathless that they cannot complete relatively short sentences in one breath
Wheeze	This can be audible wheeze or a feeling of wheeze. Very severe airway obstruction is silent (no air can move)
Widespread rash or blistering	Any discharging or blistering eruption covering more than 10% body surface area
Significant history of allergy	A known sensitivity with severe reaction (e.g. to nuts or bee sting) is significant
Local inflammation	Local inflammation will involve pain, swelling and redness confined to a particular site or area

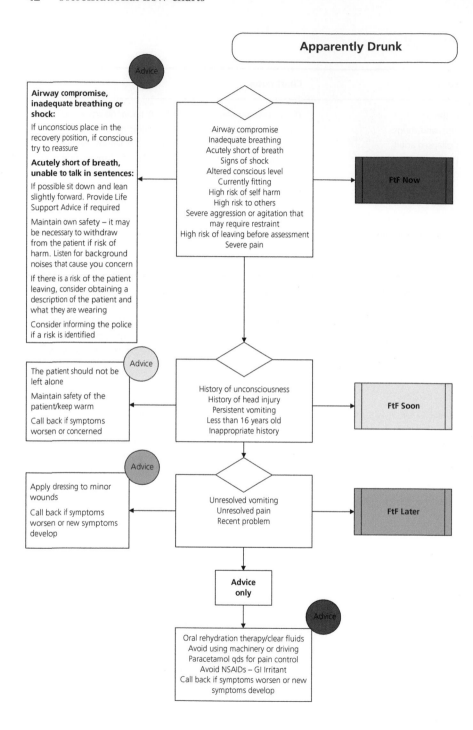

Apparently Drunk

Advice

Airway compromise, inadequate breathing or shock:

If unconscious place in the recovery position, if conscious try to reassure

Acutely short of breath, unable to talk in sentences:

If possible sit down and lean slightly forward. Provide Life Support Advice if required

Maintain own safety – it may be necessary to withdraw from the patient if risk of harm. Listen for background noises that cause you concern

If there is a risk of the patient leaving, consider obtaining a description of the patient and what they are wearing

Consider informing the police if a risk is identified

Airway compromise
Inadequate breathing
Acutely short of breath
Signs of shock
Altered conscious level
Currently fitting
High risk of self harm
High risk to others
Severe aggression or agitation that may require restraint
High risk of leaving before assessment
Severe pain

FtF Now

Advice

The patient should not be left alone

Maintain safety of the patient/keep warm

Call back if symptoms worsen or concerned

History of unconsciousness
History of head injury
Persistent vomiting
Less than 16 years old
Inappropriate history

FtF Soon

Advice

Apply dressing to minor wounds

Call back if symptoms worsen or new symptoms develop

Unresolved vomiting
Unresolved pain
Recent problem

FtF Later

Advice only

Advice

Oral rehydration therapy/clear fluids
Avoid using machinery or driving
Paracetamol qds for pain control
Avoid NSAIDs – GI Irritant
Call back if symptoms worsen or new symptoms develop

Apparently drunk

See also	Chart notes
Behaving strangely Collapsed adult Head injury	This is a presentation-defined flow diagram. A large number of patients access emergency care in an apparently drunken state. This chart implicitly recognises that not all these patients are drunk and is designed to ensure accurate identification and prioritisation of patients who are suffering from conditions which make them appear drunk, or from such severe drunkenness that their life is threatened. A number of general discriminators have been used including *Life Threat* and *Conscious Level*

Specific discriminators	Explanation
Severe aggression or agitation that may require restraint	Aggression and agitation of such a degree that restraint may be required at short notice to manage the risk of harm to self or others
High risk of leaving before assessment	Active, credible threats to leave prior to assessment pose a high risk
History of unconsciousness	There may be a reliable witness who can state whether the patient was unconscious (and for how long). If not a patient who is unable to remember the incident should be assumed to have been unconscious
History of head injury	A history of a recent physically traumatic event involving the head. Usually this will be reported by the patient, but if the patient has been unconscious, this history should be sought from a reliable witness
Persistent vomiting	Vomiting that is continuous or that occurs without any respite between episodes
Inappropriate history	When the history (story) given does not explain the physical findings, it is termed inappropriate. This is important as it is a marker of safeguarding concerns in both adults and children

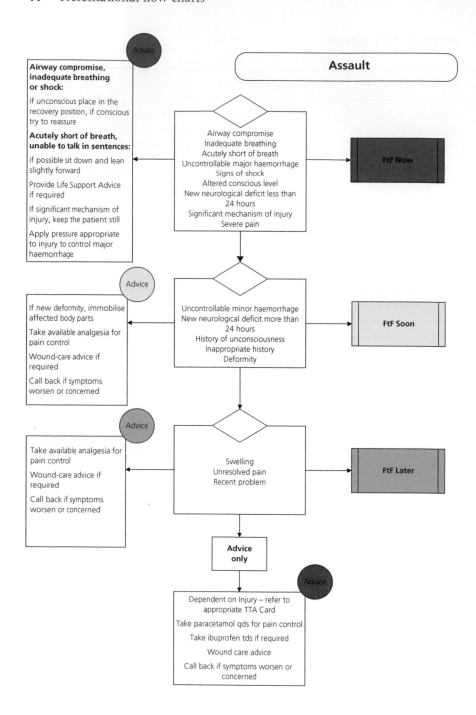

Assault

Airway compromise, inadequate breathing or shock:

if unconscious place in the recovery position, if conscious try to reassure

Acutely short of breath, unable to talk in sentences:

if possible sit down and lean slightly forward

Provide Life Support Advice if required

If significant mechanism of injury, keep the patient still

Apply pressure appropriate to injury to control major haemorrhage

Advice

Airway compromise
Inadequate breathing
Acutely short of breath
Uncontrollable major haemorrhage
Signs of shock
Altered conscious level
New neurological deficit less than 24 hours
Significant mechanism of injury
Severe pain

FtF Now

Advice

If new deformity, immobilise affected body parts

Take available analgesia for pain control

Wound-care advice if required

Call back if symptoms worsen or concerned

Uncontrollable minor haemorrhage
New neurological deficit more than 24 hours
History of unconsciousness
Inappropriate history
Deformity

FtF Soon

Advice

Take available analgesia for pain control

Wound-care advice if required

Call back if symptoms worsen or concerned

Swelling
Unresolved pain
Recent problem

FtF Later

Advice only

Advice

Dependent on Injury – refer to appropriate TTA Card

Take paracetamol qds for pain control

Take ibuprofen tds if required

Wound care advice

Call back if symptoms worsen or concerned

Assault

See also	Chart notes
Head injury Torso injury Wounds	This is a presentation-defined flow diagram. Assault is a common presentation, and patients with non-specific conditions following assault may be triaged using this chart. Patients who have specific injuries are better triaged using the charts which pertain to those injuries. A number of general discriminators are used including *Life Threat*, *Haemorrhage* and *Pain*. Specific discriminators are included to identify patients who have a significant history of injury which may indicate a more urgent requirement for treatment

Specific discriminators	Explanation
Acutely short of breath	Shortness of breath that comes on suddenly or a sudden exacerbation of chronic shortness of breath
New neurological deficit less than 24 hours	Any loss of neurological function that has come on within the previous 24 hours. This might include altered or lost sensation, weakness of the limbs (either transiently or permanently) and alterations in bladder or bowel function
Significant mechanism of injury	Penetrating injuries (stab or gunshot) and injuries with high energy transfer
New neurological deficit more than 24 hours	Any loss of neurological function including altered or lost sensation, weakness of the limbs (either transiently or permanently) and alterations in bladder or bowel function
History of unconsciousness	There may be a reliable witness who can state whether the patient was unconscious (and for how long). If not, a patient who is unable to remember the incident should be assumed to have been unconscious
Inappropriate history	When the history (story) given does not explain the physical findings, it is termed inappropriate. This is important as it is a marker of safeguarding concerns in both adults and children
Deformity	This will always be subjective. Abnormal angulation or rotation is implied
Swelling	An abnormal increase in size

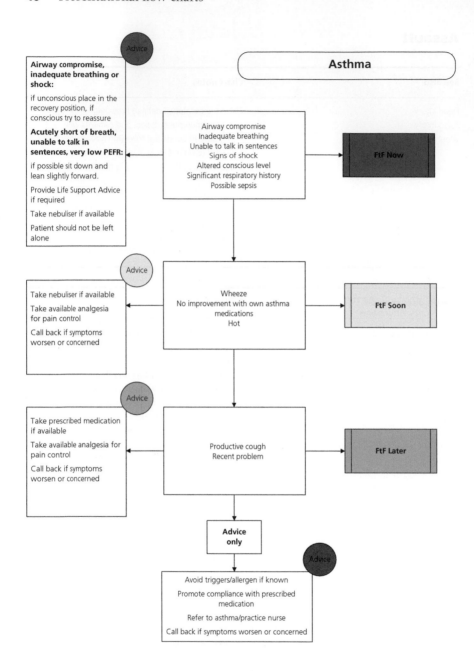

Asthma

Airway compromise, inadequate breathing or shock:

if unconscious place in the recovery position, if conscious try to reassure

Acutely short of breath, unable to talk in sentences, very low PEFR:

if possible sit down and lean slightly forward.

Provide Life Support Advice if required

Take nebuliser if available

Patient should not be left alone

Airway compromise
Inadequate breathing
Unable to talk in sentences
Signs of shock
Altered conscious level
Significant respiratory history
Possible sepsis

FtF Now

Take nebuliser if available

Take available analgesia for pain control

Call back if symptoms worsen or concerned

Wheeze
No improvement with own asthma medications
Hot

FtF Soon

Take prescribed medication if available

Take available analgesia for pain control

Call back if symptoms worsen or concerned

Productive cough
Recent problem

FtF Later

Advice only

Avoid triggers/allergen if known

Promote compliance with prescribed medication

Refer to asthma/practice nurse

Call back if symptoms worsen or concerned

Asthma

See also	Chart notes
Allergy Shortness of breath in adults Shortness of breath in children	This is a presentation-defined flow diagram which is intended for use in patients who present with the symptoms and signs of known asthma. The severity of asthmatic patients at presentation varies from those whose lives are threatened to those requiring a repeat prescription of inhalers. A number of general discriminators are used including *Life Threat* and *Conscious Level*. Specific discriminators are included to indicate those signs and symptoms which indicate severe and life-threatening asthma

Specific discriminators	Explanation
Unable to talk in sentences	Patients who are so breathless that they cannot complete relatively short sentences in one breath
Significant respiratory history	A history of previous life threatening episodes of a respiratory condition (e.g. COPD) is significant as is brittle asthma
Possible sepsis	Suspected sepsis in patients who present with altered mental state, low blood pressure (Systolic less than 100) or raised respiratory rate (rate more than 22). In children, age specific physiological tools should be used to determine if possibly septic
Wheeze	This can be audible wheeze or a feeling of wheeze. Very severe airway obstruction is silent (no air can move)
No improvement with own asthma medications	This history should be available from the patient. A failure to improve with bronchodilator therapy given by the GP or paramedic is equally significant
Productive cough	A cough which is productive of phlegm, whatever the colour

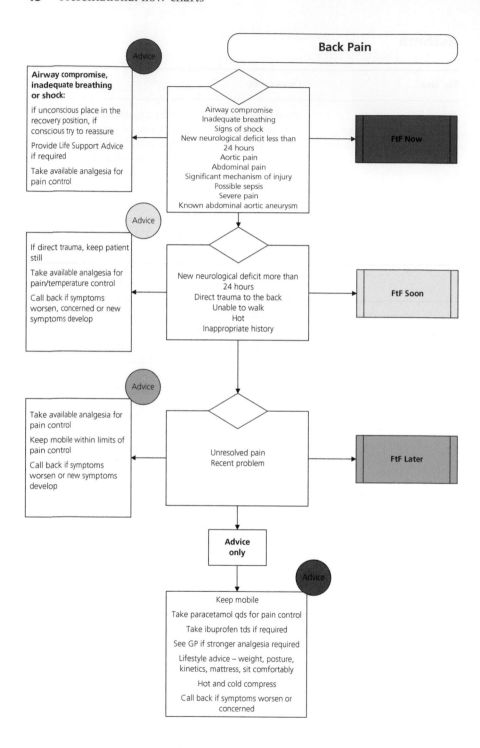

Back Pain

Airway compromise, inadequate breathing or shock:

if unconscious place in the recovery position, if conscious try to reassure

Provide Life Support Advice if required

Take available analgesia for pain control

Airway compromise
Inadequate breathing
Signs of shock
New neurological deficit less than 24 hours
Aortic pain
Abdominal pain
Significant mechanism of injury
Possible sepsis
Severe pain
Known abdominal aortic aneurysm

FtF Now

If direct trauma, keep patient still

Take available analgesia for pain/temperature control

Call back if symptoms worsen, concerned or new symptoms develop

New neurological deficit more than 24 hours
Direct trauma to the back
Unable to walk
Hot
Inappropriate history

FtF Soon

Take available analgesia for pain control

Keep mobile within limits of pain control

Call back if symptoms worsen or new symptoms develop

Unresolved pain
Recent problem

FtF Later

Advice only

Keep mobile

Take paracetamol qds for pain control

Take ibuprofen tds if required

See GP if stronger analgesia required

Lifestyle advice – weight, posture, kinetics, mattress, sit comfortably

Hot and cold compress

Call back if symptoms worsen or concerned

Back pain

See also	Chart notes
Abdominal pain Neck pain	This is a presentation-defined flow diagram. Patients with back pain may present either as an acute event or as an acute exacerbation of a chronic problem. A number of general discriminators are used including *Life Threat*, *Pain* and *Temperature*. Specific discriminators have been selected in order to allow for appropriate categorisation of more urgent problems. In particular, discriminators are included to allow appropriate classification of abdominal aneurysm and patients with neurological signs and symptoms

Specific discriminators	Explanation
New neurological deficit less than 24 hours	Any loss of neurological function that has come on within the previous 24 hours. This might include altered or lost sensation, weakness of the limbs (either transiently or permanently) and alterations in bladder or bowel function
Abdominal pain	Any pain felt in the abdomen. Abdominal pain associated with back pain may indicate abdominal aortic aneurysm, whilst association with PV bleeding may indicate ectopic pregnancy or miscarriage
Significant mechanism of injury	Penetrating injuries (stab or gunshot) and injuries with high energy transfer
Possible sepsis	Suspected sepsis in patients who present with altered mental state, low blood pressure (Systolic less than 100) or raised respiratory rate (rate more than 22). In children, age specific physiological tools should be used to determine if possibly septic
Aortic pain	The onset of symptoms is sudden and the leading symptom is severe abdominal or chest pain. The pain may be described as sharp, stabbing or ripping in character. Classically aortic chest pain is felt around the sternum and then radiates to the shoulder blades, aortic abdominal pain is felt in the centre of the abdomen and radiates to the back. The pain may get better or even vanish and then recur elsewhere. Over time, pain may also be felt in the arms, neck, lower jaw, stomach or hips
New neurological deficit more than 24 hours	Any loss of neurological function including altered or lost sensation, weakness of the limbs (either transiently or permanently) and alterations in bladder or bowel function
Direct trauma to the back	This may be top to bottom (loading) for instance when people fall and land on their feet, bending (forwards, backwards or to the side) or twisting
Unable to walk	It is important to try and distinguish between patients who have pain and difficulty walking and those who *cannot* walk. Only the latter can be said to be unable to walk
Inappropriate history	When the history (story) given does not explain the physical findings, it is termed inappropriate. This is important as it is a marker of safeguarding concerns in both adults and children

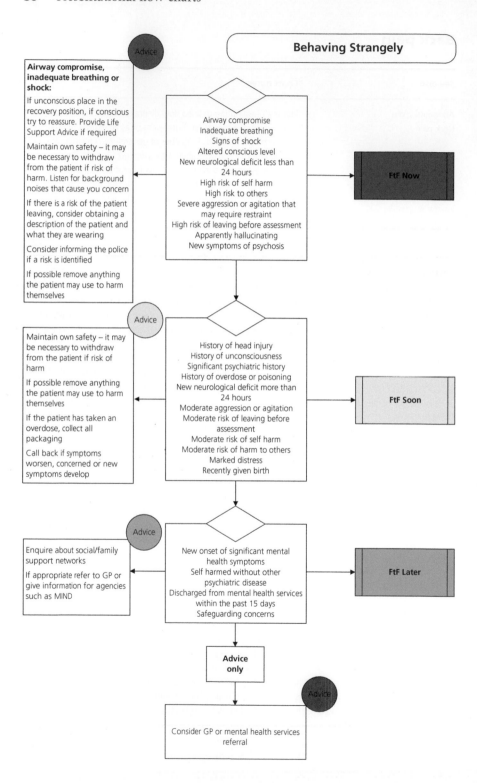

Behaving Strangely

Airway compromise, inadequate breathing or shock:

If unconscious place in the recovery position, if conscious try to reassure. Provide Life Support Advice if required

Maintain own safety – it may be necessary to withdraw from the patient if risk of harm. Listen for background noises that cause you concern

If there is a risk of the patient leaving, consider obtaining a description of the patient and what they are wearing

Consider informing the police if a risk is identified

If possible remove anything the patient may use to harm themselves

Airway compromise
Inadequate breathing
Signs of shock
Altered conscious level
New neurological deficit less than 24 hours
High risk of self harm
High risk to others
Severe aggression or agitation that may require restraint
High risk of leaving before assessment
Apparently hallucinating
New symptoms of psychosis

FtF Now

Maintain own safety – it may be necessary to withdraw from the patient if risk of harm

If possible remove anything the patient may use to harm themselves

If the patient has taken an overdose, collect all packaging

Call back if symptoms worsen, concerned or new symptoms develop

History of head injury
History of unconsciousness
Significant psychiatric history
History of overdose or poisoning
New neurological deficit more than 24 hours
Moderate aggression or agitation
Moderate risk of leaving before assessment
Moderate risk of self harm
Moderate risk of harm to others
Marked distress
Recently given birth

FtF Soon

Enquire about social/family support networks

If appropriate refer to GP or give information for agencies such as MIND

New onset of significant mental health symptoms
Self harmed without other psychiatric disease
Discharged from mental health services within the past 15 days
Safeguarding concerns

FtF Later

Advice only

Consider GP or mental health services referral

Behaving strangely

See also	Chart notes
Apparently drunk Mental illness	This is a presentation-defined flow diagram. Patients who behave strangely may have either a psychiatric or a physical cause for their presentation. This chart is designed to allow the accurate prioritisation of both these groups of patients. A number of general discriminators have been used including *Life Threat* and *Conscious Level*. Specific discriminators are used and in particular the concepts of risk of harm to others and risks of self-harm are introduced

Specific discriminators	Explanation
New neurological deficit less than 24 hours	Any loss of neurological function that has come on within the previous 24 hours. This might include altered or lost sensation, weakness of the limbs (either transiently or permanently) and alterations in bladder or bowel function
High risk of self harm	An initial view of the risk of harm to self can be formed by considering the patient's behaviour. Patients who are threatening to harm themselves and who are actively seeking the means to do so are at high risk
High risk to others	An initial view of the risk of harm to others can be judged by assessing posture (tense, clenched), speech (loud, using threatening words) loud background noise can be an indicator and motor behaviour (restless, pacing, lunging at others). High risk should be assumed if weapons and potential victims are available and no controls are already in place
Apparently hallucinating	Patients who are apparently hallucinating may appear distracted and may appear to react to stimuli (primarily visual and auditory) that are not apparent to anyone else
History of head injury	A history of a recent physically traumatic event involving the head. Usually this will be reported by the patient, but if the patient has been unconscious, this history should be sought from a reliable witness
History of unconsciousness	There may be a reliable witness who can state whether the patient was unconscious (and for how long). If not, a patient who is unable to remember the incident should be assumed to have been unconscious
Significant psychiatric history	A history of a major psychiatric illness or event
History of overdose or poisoning	This information may come from others or may be deduced if medication is missing
New neurological deficit more than 24 hours	Any loss of neurological function including altered or lost sensation, weakness of the limbs (either transiently or permanently) and alterations in bladder or bowel function
Recently given birth	A woman who has given birth within the past 3 months

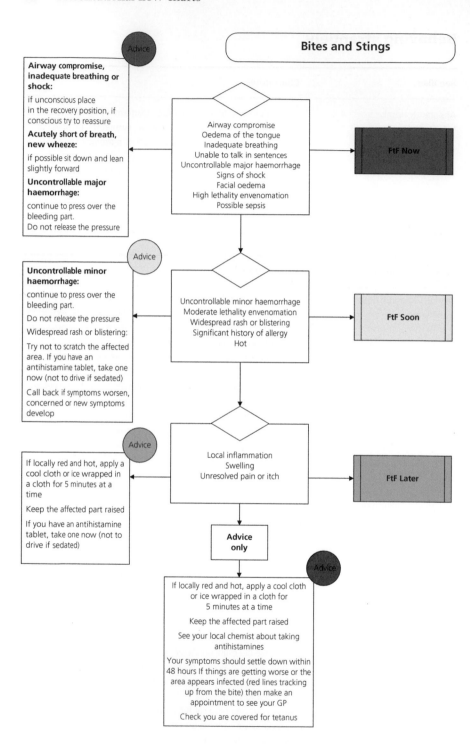

Bites and Stings

Advice

Airway compromise, inadequate breathing or shock:

if unconscious place in the recovery position, if conscious try to reassure

Acutely short of breath, new wheeze:

if possible sit down and lean slightly forward

Uncontrollable major haemorrhage:

continue to press over the bleeding part.
Do not release the pressure

Airway compromise
Oedema of the tongue
Inadequate breathing
Unable to talk in sentences
Uncontrollable major haemorrhage
Signs of shock
Facial oedema
High lethality envenomation
Possible sepsis

FtF Now

Advice

Uncontrollable minor haemorrhage:

continue to press over the bleeding part.

Do not release the pressure

Widespread rash or blistering:

Try not to scratch the affected area. If you have an antihistamine tablet, take one now (not to drive if sedated)

Call back if symptoms worsen, concerned or new symptoms develop

Uncontrollable minor haemorrhage
Moderate lethality envenomation
Widespread rash or blistering
Significant history of allergy
Hot

FtF Soon

Advice

If locally red and hot, apply a cool cloth or ice wrapped in a cloth for 5 minutes at a time

Keep the affected part raised

If you have an antihistamine tablet, take one now (not to drive if sedated)

Local inflammation
Swelling
Unresolved pain or itch

FtF Later

Advice only

Advice

If locally red and hot, apply a cool cloth or ice wrapped in a cloth for 5 minutes at a time

Keep the affected part raised

See your local chemist about taking antihistamines

Your symptoms should settle down within 48 hours If things are getting worse or the area appears infected (red lines tracking up from the bite) then make an appointment to see your GP

Check you are covered for tetanus

Bites and stings

See also	Chart notes
Abscesses and local infections Allergy	This is a presentation-defined flow diagram designed to allow accurate prioritisation of patients who present following bites and stings. Bites may, of course, range from those delivered by insects to those delivered by large animals; therefore there is a complete range of priority covered by this presentation. A number of general discriminators are used including *Life Threat*, *Haemorrhage* and *Pain*. Specific discriminators have been added to the chart to allow accurate identification of patients who need immediate treatment because of more severe injury or the development of allergic reactions

Specific discriminators	Explanation
Oedema of the tongue	Swelling of the tongue of any degree
Unable to talk in sentences	Patients who are so breathless that they cannot complete relatively short sentences in one breath
Facial oedema	Diffuse swelling around the face usually involving the lips
High lethality envenomation	Lethality is the potential of the envenomation to cause harm. Local knowledge may allow identification of the venomous creature, but advice may be required. If in doubt, assume a high risk
Possible sepsis	Suspected sepsis in patients who present with altered mental state, low blood pressure (Systolic less than 100) or raised respiratory rate (rate more than 22). In children, age specific physiological tools should be used to determine if possibly septic
Moderate lethality envenomation	Lethality is the potential of the envenomation to cause harm. Local knowledge may allow identification of the venomous creature, but advice may be required
Widespread rash or blistering	Any discharging or blistering eruption covering more than 10% body surface area
Significant history of allergy	A known sensitivity with severe reaction (e.g. to nuts or bee sting) is significant
Local inflammation	Local inflammation will involve pain, swelling and redness confined to a particular site or area

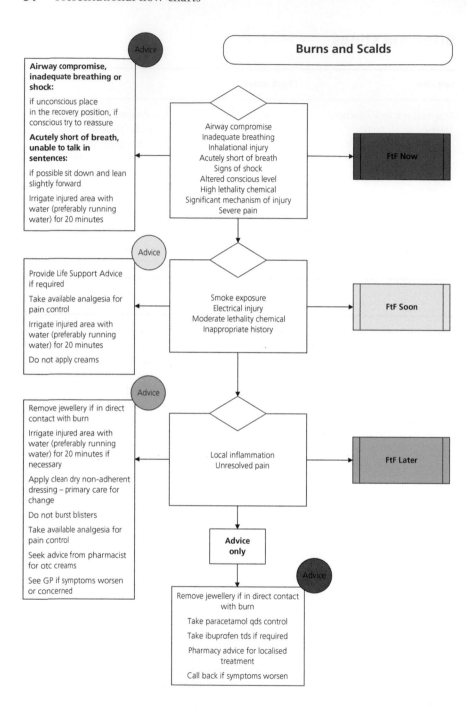

Burns and Scalds

Airway compromise, inadequate breathing or shock:

if unconscious place in the recovery position, if conscious try to reassure

Acutely short of breath, unable to talk in sentences:

if possible sit down and lean slightly forward

Irrigate injured area with water (preferably running water) for 20 minutes

Advice

Airway compromise
Inadequate breathing
Inhalational injury
Acutely short of breath
Signs of shock
Altered conscious level
High lethality chemical
Significant mechanism of injury
Severe pain

FtF Now

Provide Life Support Advice if required

Take available analgesia for pain control

Irrigate injured area with water (preferably running water) for 20 minutes

Do not apply creams

Advice

Smoke exposure
Electrical injury
Moderate lethality chemical
Inappropriate history

FtF Soon

Remove jewellery if in direct contact with burn

Irrigate injured area with water (preferably running water) for 20 minutes if necessary

Apply clean dry non-adherent dressing – primary care for change

Do not burst blisters

Take available analgesia for pain control

Seek advice from pharmacist for otc creams

See GP if symptoms worsen or concerned

Advice

Local inflammation
Unresolved pain

FtF Later

Advice only

Advice

Remove jewellery if in direct contact with burn

Take paracetamol qds control

Take ibuprofen tds if required

Pharmacy advice for localised treatment

Call back if symptoms worsen

Burns and scalds

	Chart notes
	This is a presentation-defined flow diagram. There is a complete range of severity with this presentation and the chart has been designed to allow accurate identification of patients within each category. A number of general discriminators are used including *Life Threat*, *Conscious Level* and *Pain*. Specific discriminators have been added to allow identification of patients who have suffered inhalational injury and those in whom the mechanism suggests that further investigation and treatment may be appropriate

Specific discriminators	Explanation
Inhalational injury	A history of being confined in a smoke-filled space is the most reliable indicator of smoke inhalation. Carbon deposits around the mouth and nose and hoarse voice may present. History is also the most reliable way of diagnosing inhalation of chemicals – there will not necessarily be any signs
Acutely short of breath	Shortness of breath that comes on suddenly or a sudden exacerbation of chronic shortness of breath
High lethality chemical	Lethality is the potential of the chemical to cause harm. Advice may be required to establish the level of risk. If in doubt, assume a high risk
Significant mechanism of injury	Penetrating injuries (stab or gunshot) and injuries with high energy transfer
Smoke exposure	Smoke inhalation should be assumed if the patient has been confined in a smoke-filled space. Physical signs such as oral or nasal soot are less reliable but significant if present
Electrical injury	Any injury caused or possibly caused by electric current. This includes AC and DC and both artificial and natural sources
Moderate lethality chemical	Lethality is the potential of the chemical to cause harm. Advice may be required to establish the level of risk. If in doubt, assume a high risk
Inappropriate history	When the history (story) given does not explain the physical findings, it is termed inappropriate. This is important as it is a marker of safeguarding concerns in both adults and children
Local inflammation	Local inflammation will involve pain, swelling and redness confined to a particular site or area

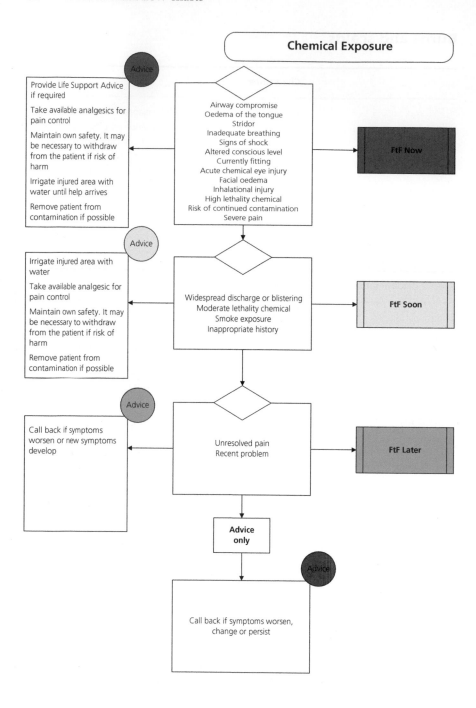

Chemical Exposure

Advice

Provide Life Support Advice if required

Take available analgesics for pain control

Maintain own safety. It may be necessary to withdraw from the patient if risk of harm

Irrigate injured area with water until help arrives

Remove patient from contamination if possible

Airway compromise
Oedema of the tongue
Stridor
Inadequate breathing
Signs of shock
Altered conscious level
Currently fitting
Acute chemical eye injury
Facial oedema
Inhalational injury
High lethality chemical
Risk of continued contamination
Severe pain

FtF Now

Advice

Irrigate injured area with water

Take available analgesic for pain control

Maintain own safety. It may be necessary to withdraw from the patient if risk of harm

Remove patient from contamination if possible

Widespread discharge or blistering
Moderate lethality chemical
Smoke exposure
Inappropriate history

FtF Soon

Advice

Call back if symptoms worsen or new symptoms develop

Unresolved pain
Recent problem

FtF Later

Advice
only

Advice

Call back if symptoms worsen, change or persist

Chemical exposure

See also	Chart notes
Overdose and poisoning Shortness of breath in adults Shortness of breath in children	This is a presentation-defined flow diagram. While this presentation is not common, it is important because it is often the chief complaint of the patient. The signs and symptoms do not necessarily fit easily into any other presentational group. A number of general discriminators are used including *Life Threat, Conscious Level* and *Pain*. Specific discriminators which include those for the shortness of breath have been added to appropriate categories. *Acute Chemical Eye Injury* and *Risk of Continued Contamination* appear in the 'face to face Now' category

Specific discriminators	Explanation
Oedema of the tongue	Swelling of the tongue of any degree
Stridor	This may be an inspiratory or expiratory noise or both. Stridor is heard best on breathing with the mouth open
Acute chemical eye injury	Any substance splashed into or placed into the eye within the past 12 hours that caused stinging, burning or reduced vision should be assumed to be have caused chemical injury
Facial oedema	Diffuse swelling around the face usually involving the lips
Inhalational injury	A history of being confined in a smoke filled space is the most reliable indicator of smoke inhalation. Carbon deposits around the mouth and nose and hoarse voice may be present. History is also the most reliable way of diagnosing inhalation of chemicals – there will not necessarily be any signs
High lethality chemical	Lethality is the potential of the chemical to cause harm. Advice may be required to establish the level of risk. If in doubt, assume high risk
Risk of continued contamination	If chemical exposure is likely to continue (usually due to lack of adequate decontamination), then this discriminator applies. Risks to health care workers must not be forgotten if this situation occurs
Widespread discharge or blistering	Any discharging or blistering eruption covering more than 10% body surface area
Moderate lethality chemical	Lethality is the potential of the chemical to cause harm. Advice may be required to establish the level of risk. If in doubt, assume high risk
Smoke exposure	Smoke inhalation should be assumed if the patient has been confined in a smoke-filled space. Physical signs such as oral or nasal soot are less reliable but significant if present
Inappropriate history	When the history (story) given does not explain the physical findings, it is termed inappropriate. This is important as it is a marker of safeguarding concerns in both adults and children

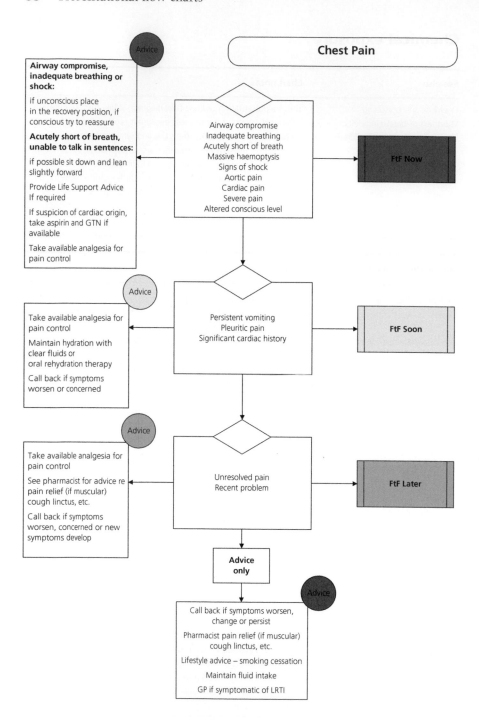

Chest Pain

Airway compromise, inadequate breathing or shock:

if unconscious place in the recovery position, if conscious try to reassure

Acutely short of breath, unable to talk in sentences:

if possible sit down and lean slightly forward

Provide Life Support Advice If required

If suspicion of cardiac origin, take aspirin and GTN if available

Take available analgesia for pain control

Airway compromise
Inadequate breathing
Acutely short of breath
Massive haemoptysis
Signs of shock
Aortic pain
Cardiac pain
Severe pain
Altered conscious level

FtF Now

Take available analgesia for pain control

Maintain hydration with clear fluids or oral rehydration therapy

Call back if symptoms worsen or concerned

Persistent vomiting
Pleuritic pain
Significant cardiac history

FtF Soon

Take available analgesia for pain control

See pharmacist for advice re pain relief (if muscular) cough linctus, etc.

Call back if symptoms worsen, concerned or new symptoms develop

Unresolved pain
Recent problem

FtF Later

Advice only

Call back if symptoms worsen, change or persist

Pharmacist pain relief (if muscular) cough linctus, etc.

Lifestyle advice – smoking cessation

Maintain fluid intake

GP if symptomatic of LRTI

Advice

Chest pain

Chart notes

This is a presentation-defined flow diagram. Chest pain is a common presentation. Causes of chest pain may vary from acute myocardial infarction to muscular irritation, and appropriate categorisation is paramount. A number of general discriminators are used including *Life Threat* and *Pain*. Specific discriminators include the nature and severity of pain (cardiac or pleuritic)

Specific discriminators	Explanation
Acutely short of breath	Shortness of breath that comes on suddenly or a sudden exacerbation of chronic shortness of breath
Massive haemoptysis	Coughing up large amounts of fresh or clotted blood. Not to be confused with streaks of blood in saliva
Aortic pain	The onset of symptoms is sudden and the leading symptom is severe abdominal or chest pain. The pain may be described as sharp, stabbing or ripping in character. Classically aortic chest pain is felt around the sternum and then radiates to the shoulder blades, aortic abdominal pain is felt in the centre of the abdomen and radiates to the back. The pain may get better or even vanish and then recur elsewhere. Over time, pain may also be felt in the arms, neck, lower jaw, stomach or hips
Cardiac pain	Classically a severe dull 'gripping' or 'heavy' pain in the centre of the chest, radiating to the left arm or to the neck. May be associated with sweating and nausea
Persistent vomiting	Vomiting that is continuous or that occurs without any respite between episodes
Pleuritic pain	A sharp, localised pain in the chest that worsens on breathing, coughing or sneezing
Significant cardiac history	A known recurrent dysrhythmia which has life-threatening effects is significant, as is a known cardiac condition that may deteriorate rapidly

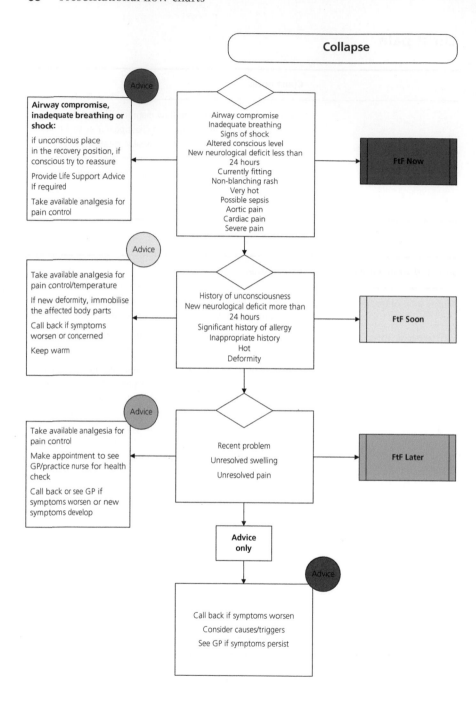

Collapse

See also	Chart notes
Apparently drunk Falls Fits Unwell adult	This is a presentation-defined flow diagram. Presentation with collapse is not uncommon and this chart is designed to allow rapid triage of patients who present in this way. A number of general discriminators are used including *Life Threat*, *Conscious Level*, *Pain* and *Temperature*. Specific discriminators have been added to the chart to try and rule out more serious pathology. As with all charts, those pathologies (such as myocardial infarction) which can potentially benefit from early intevention are deliberately categorised highly

Specific discriminators	Explanation
New neurological deficit less than 24 hours	Any loss of neurological function that has come on within the previous 24 hours. This might include altered or lost sensation, weakness of the limbs (either transiently or permanently) and alterations in bladder or bowel function
Non-blanching rash	A rash that does not blanch (go white) when pressure is applied to it. Often tested using a glass tumbler to apply pressure as any colour change can be observed through the bottom of the tumbler
Possible sepsis	Suspected sepsis in patients who present with altered mental state, low blood pressure (Systolic less than 100) or raised respiratory rate (rate more than 22). In children, age specific physiological tools should be used to determine if possibly septic
Aortic pain	The onset of symptoms is sudden and the leading symptom is severe abdominal or chest pain. The pain may be described as sharp, stabbing or ripping in character. Classically aortic chest pain is felt around the sternum and then radiates to the shoulder blades, aortic abdominal pain is felt in the centre of the abdomen and radiates to the back. The pain may get better or even vanish and then recur elsewhere. Over time, pain may also be felt in the arms, neck, lower jaw, stomach or hips
Cardiac pain	Classically a severe dull 'gripping' or 'heavy' pain in the centre of the chest, radiating to the left arm or to the neck. May be associated with sweating and nausea
New neurological deficit more than 24 hours	Any loss of neurological function including altered or lost sensation, weakness of the limbs (either transiently or permanently) and alterations in bladder or bowel function
Significant history of allergy	A known sensitivity with severe reaction (e.g. to nuts or bee sting) is significant
Inappropriate history	When the history (story) given does not explain the physical findings, it is termed inappropriate. This is important as it is a marker of safeguarding concerns in both adults and children
Deformity	This will always be subjective. Abnormal angulation or rotation is implied

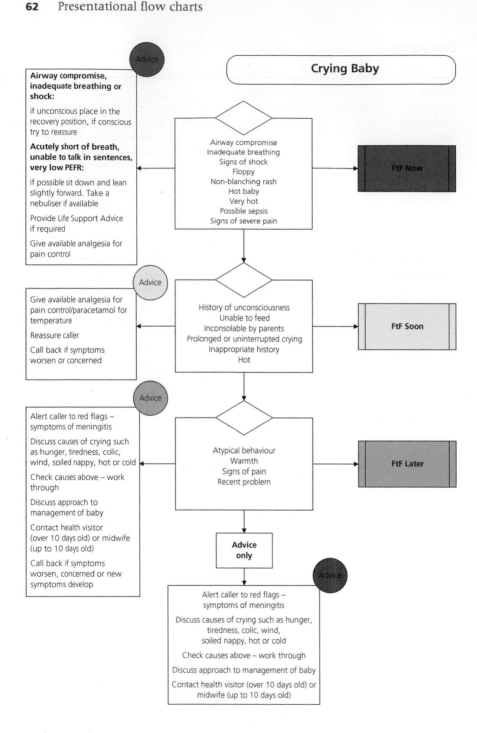

Crying Baby

Advice

Airway compromise, inadequate breathing or shock:

if unconscious place in the recovery position, if conscious try to reassure

Acutely short of breath, unable to talk in sentences, very low PEFR:

if possible sit down and lean slightly forward. Take a nebuliser if available

Provide Life Support Advice if required

Give available analgesia for pain control

Airway compromise
Inadequate breathing
Signs of shock
Floppy
Non-blanching rash
Hot baby
Very hot
Possible sepsis
Signs of severe pain

FtF Now

Advice

Give available analgesia for pain control/paracetamol for temperature

Reassure caller

Call back if symptoms worsen or concerned

History of unconsciousness
Unable to feed
Inconsolable by parents
Prolonged or uninterrupted crying
Inappropriate history
Hot

FtF Soon

Advice

Alert caller to red flags – symptoms of meningitis

Discuss causes of crying such as hunger, tiredness, colic, wind, soiled nappy, hot or cold

Check causes above – work through

Discuss approach to management of baby

Contact health visitor (over 10 days old) or midwife (up to 10 days old)

Call back if symptoms worsen, concerned or new symptoms develop

Atypical behaviour
Warmth
Signs of pain
Recent problem

FtF Later

Advice only

Advice

Alert caller to red flags – symptoms of meningitis

Discuss causes of crying such as hunger, tiredness, colic, wind, soiled nappy, hot or cold

Check causes above – work through

Discuss approach to management of baby

Contact health visitor (over 10 days old) or midwife (up to 10 days old)

Crying baby

See also	Chart notes
Unwell child Unwell newborn Worried parent	This is a presentation-defined flow diagram. This chart has been designed to allow accurate prioritisation of children who are presented by their parents with a chief complaint of crying. A number of general discriminators have been used including *Life Threat*, *Conscious Level* and *Pain*. Specific discriminators include those which allow recognition of more specific pathologies such as septicaemia or which indicate that a more serious pathology might exist. If the patient is under 28 days, the Unwell newborn chart should be used

Specific discriminators	Explanation
Floppy	Parents may describe their children as floppy. Tone is generally reduced – the most noticeable sign is often lolling of the head
Non-blanching rash	A rash that does not blanch (go white) when pressure is applied to it. Often tested using a glass tumbler to apply pressure as any colour change can be observed through the bottom of the tumbler
Possible sepsis	Suspected sepsis in patients who present with altered mental state, low blood pressure (Systolic less than 100) or raised respiratory rate (rate more than 22). In children, age specific physiological tools should be used to determine if possibly septic
Signs of severe pain	Young children and babies in severe pain cannot complain. They will usually cry out continuously and inconsolably and be tachycardic. They may well exhibit signs such as pallor and sweating
Unable to feed	This is usually reported by the parents. Children who will not take any solid or liquid (as appropriate) by mouth
Inconsolable by parents	Children whose crying or distress does not respond to attempts by their parents to comfort them fulfil this criterion
Prolonged or uninterrupted crying	A child who has cried continuously for 2 hours or more fulfils this criteria
Inappropriate history	When the history (story) given does not explain the physical findings, it is termed inappropriate. This is important as it is a marker of safeguarding concerns in both adults and children
Atypical behaviour	A child who behaves in a way that is not usual in the given situation. The carers will often volunteer this information. Such children are often referred to as fractious or 'out of sorts'

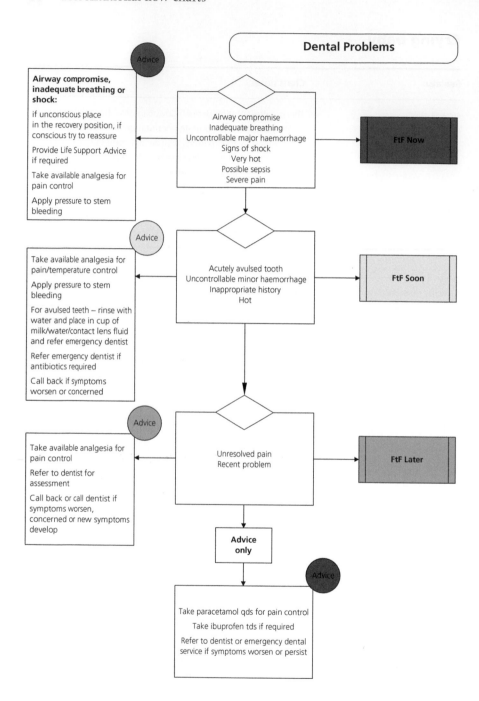

Dental Problems

Advice

Airway compromise, inadequate breathing or shock:

if unconscious place in the recovery position, if conscious try to reassure

Provide Life Support Advice if required

Take available analgesia for pain control

Apply pressure to stem bleeding

Airway compromise
Inadequate breathing
Uncontrollable major haemorrhage
Signs of shock
Very hot
Possible sepsis
Severe pain

FtF Now

Advice

Take available analgesia for pain/temperature control

Apply pressure to stem bleeding

For avulsed teeth – rinse with water and place in cup of milk/water/contact lens fluid and refer emergency dentist

Refer emergency dentist if antibiotics required

Call back if symptoms worsen or concerned

Acutely avulsed tooth
Uncontrollable minor haemorrhage
Inappropriate history
Hot

FtF Soon

Advice

Take available analgesia for pain control

Refer to dentist for assessment

Call back or call dentist if symptoms worsen, concerned or new symptoms develop

Unresolved pain
Recent problem

FtF Later

**Advice
only**

Advice

Take paracetamol qds for pain control

Take ibuprofen tds if required

Refer to dentist or emergency dental service if symptoms worsen or persist

Dental problems

See also	Chart notes
Facial problems	This is a presentation-defined flow diagram designed to allow accurate prioritisation of patients presenting problems affecting teeth or gums. A number of general discriminators have been used including *Life Threat*, *Pain*, *Haemorrhage* and *Temperature*. Acute avulsion of a tooth has been included in the very urgent 'face to face Soon' category since speed of reimplantation affects outcome

Specific discriminators	Explanation
Possible sepsis	Suspected sepsis in patients who present with altered mental state, low blood pressure (Systolic less than 100) or raised respiratory rate (rate more than 22). In children, age specific physiological tools should be used to determine if possibly septic
Acutely avulsed tooth	A tooth that has been avulsed intact within the previous 24 hours
Inappropriate history	When the history (story) given does not explain the physical findings, it is termed inappropriate. This is important as it is a marker of safeguarding concerns in both adults and children

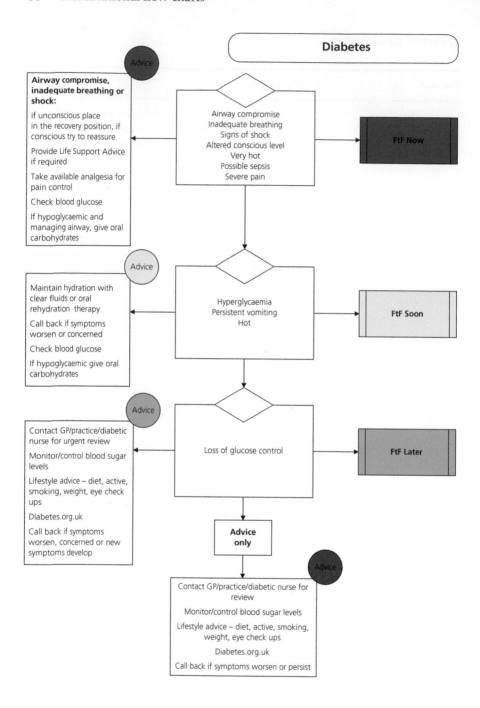

Diabetes

Airway compromise, inadequate breathing or shock:

if unconscious place in the recovery position, if conscious try to reassure

Provide Life Support Advice if required

Take available analgesia for pain control

Check blood glucose

If hypoglycaemic and managing airway, give oral carbohydrates

Advice

Airway compromise
Inadequate breathing
Signs of shock
Altered conscious level
Very hot
Possible sepsis
Severe pain

FtF Now

Maintain hydration with clear fluids or oral rehydration therapy

Call back if symptoms worsen or concerned

Check blood glucose

If hypoglycaemic give oral carbohydrates

Advice

Hyperglycaemia
Persistent vomiting
Hot

FtF Soon

Contact GP/practice/diabetic nurse for urgent review

Monitor/control blood sugar levels

Lifestyle advice – diet, active, smoking, weight, eye check ups

Diabetes.org.uk

Call back if symptoms worsen, concerned or new symptoms develop

Advice

Loss of glucose control

FtF Later

Advice only

Advice

Contact GP/practice/diabetic nurse for review

Monitor/control blood sugar levels

Lifestyle advice – diet, active, smoking, weight, eye check ups

Diabetes.org.uk

Call back if symptoms worsen or persist

Diabetes

	Chart notes
	This is a presentation-defined flow diagram designed to allow categorisation of known diabetic patients. A number of general discriminators are used including *Life Threat*, *Conscious Level*, *Blood Glucose Level* and *Temperature*. If the patient is under 28 days, the Unwell newborn chart should be used

Specific discriminators	Explanation
Possible sepsis	Suspected sepsis in patients who present with altered mental state, low blood pressure (Systolic less than 100) or raised respiratory rate (rate more than 22). In children, age specific physiological tools should be used to determine if possibly septic
Hyperglycaemia	Glucose greater than 17 mmol/l

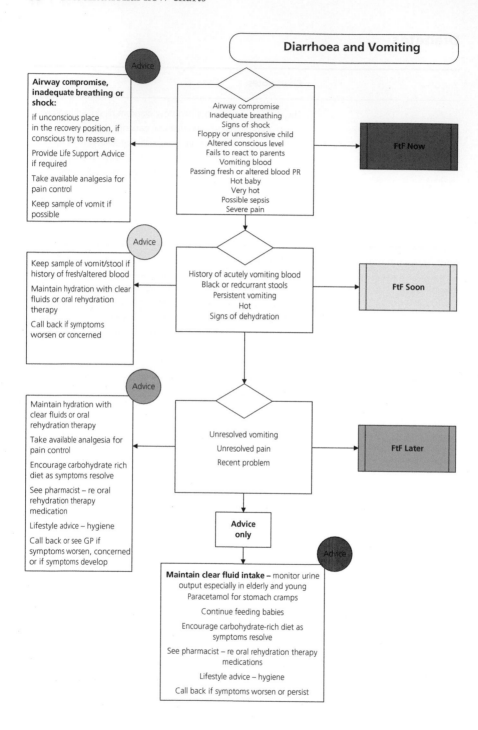

Diarrhoea and Vomiting

Advice

Airway compromise, inadequate breathing or shock:

if unconscious place in the recovery position, if conscious try to reassure

Provide Life Support Advice if required

Take available analgesia for pain control

Keep sample of vomit if possible

Airway compromise
Inadequate breathing
Signs of shock
Floppy or unresponsive child
Altered conscious level
Fails to react to parents
Vomiting blood
Passing fresh or altered blood PR
Hot baby
Very hot
Possible sepsis
Severe pain

FtF Now

Advice

Keep sample of vomit/stool if history of fresh/altered blood

Maintain hydration with clear fluids or oral rehydration therapy

Call back if symptoms worsen or concerned

History of acutely vomiting blood
Black or redcurrant stools
Persistent vomiting
Hot
Signs of dehydration

FtF Soon

Advice

Maintain hydration with clear fluids or oral rehydration therapy

Take available analgesia for pain control

Encourage carbohydrate rich diet as symptoms resolve

See pharmacist – re oral rehydration therapy medication

Lifestyle advice – hygiene

Call back or see GP if symptoms worsen, concerned or if symptoms develop

Unresolved vomiting

Unresolved pain

Recent problem

FtF Later

Advice only

Advice

Maintain clear fluid intake – monitor urine output especially in elderly and young
Paracetamol for stomach cramps

Continue feeding babies

Encourage carbohydrate-rich diet as symptoms resolve

See pharmacist – re oral rehydration therapy medications

Lifestyle advice – hygiene

Call back if symptoms worsen or persist

Diarrhoea and vomiting

See also	Chart notes
Abdominal pain in adults Abdominal pain in children GI bleeding	This is a presentation-defined flow diagram. Most patients who present with diarrhoea or vomiting do not have high priority. However, a number may have serious underlying pathology. A number of general discriminators are used including *Life Threat* and *Pain*. Specific discriminators have been included to ensure that patients suffering from GI bleeding and those with dehydration and other severe effects of diarrhoea and vomiting are included in the appropriate categories

Specific discriminators	Explanation
Floppy	Parents may describe their children as floppy. Tone is generally reduced – the most noticeable sign is often lolling of the head
Fails to react to parents	Failure to react in any way to a parents' face or voice. Abnormal reactions and apparent lack of recognition of a parent are also worrying signs
Vomiting blood	Vomited blood may be fresh (bright or dark red) or coffee ground in appearance
Passing fresh or altered blood PR	In active massive GI bleeding, dark red blood will be passed PR. As GI transit time increases, this becomes darker, eventually becoming melaena
Possible sepsis	Suspected sepsis in patients who present with altered mental state, low blood pressure (Systolic less than 100) or raised respiratory rate (rate more than 22). In children, age specific physiological tools should be used to determine if possibly septic
History of acutely vomiting blood	Frank haematemesis, vomiting of altered blood (coffee ground) or of blood mixed in the vomit within the past 24 hours
Black or redcurrant stools	Any blackness fulfils the criteria of black stool while a dark red stool, classically seen in intussusceptions, is redcurrant stool
Persistent vomiting	Vomiting that is continuous or that occurs without any respite between episodes
Signs of dehydration	These include dry tongue, sunken eyes, decreased skin turgor and, in small babies, a sunken anterior fontanelle. Usually associated with a low urine output

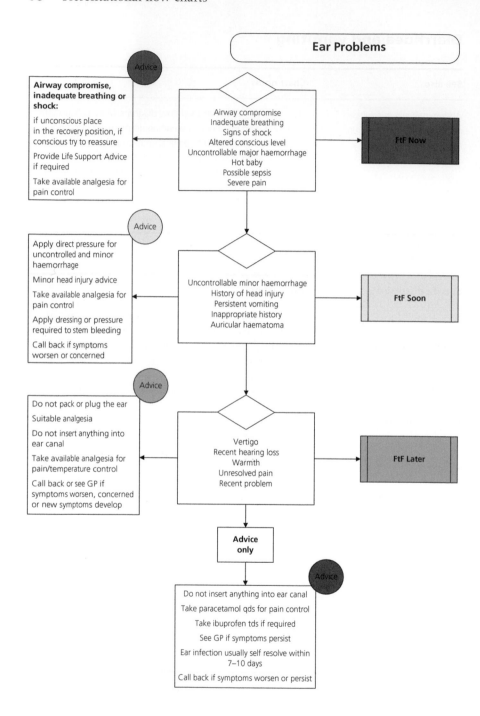

Ear Problems

Advice

Airway compromise, inadequate breathing or shock:

if unconscious place in the recovery position, if conscious try to reassure

Provide Life Support Advice if required

Take available analgesia for pain control

Airway compromise
Inadequate breathing
Signs of shock
Altered conscious level
Uncontrollable major haemorrhage
Hot baby
Possible sepsis
Severe pain

FtF Now

Advice

Apply direct pressure for uncontrolled and minor haemorrhage

Minor head injury advice

Take available analgesia for pain control

Apply dressing or pressure required to stem bleeding

Call back if symptoms worsen or concerned

Uncontrollable minor haemorrhage
History of head injury
Persistent vomiting
Inappropriate history
Auricular haematoma

FtF Soon

Advice

Do not pack or plug the ear

Suitable analgesia

Do not insert anything into ear canal

Take available analgesia for pain/temperature control

Call back or see GP if symptoms worsen, concerned or new symptoms develop

Vertigo
Recent hearing loss
Warmth
Unresolved pain
Recent problem

FtF Later

Advice only

Advice

Do not insert anything into ear canal

Take paracetamol qds for pain control

Take ibuprofen tds if required

See GP if symptoms persist

Ear infection usually self resolve within 7–10 days

Call back if symptoms worsen or persist

Ear problems

See also	Chart notes
Facial problems Head injury	This is a presentation-defined flow diagram designed to allow accurate prioritisation of patients presenting with conditions affecting the ear. A number of general discriminators are used including *Life Threat*, *Pain*, *Haemorrhage* and *Temperature*. If the patient is under 28 days, the Unwell newborn chart should be used

Specific discriminators	Explanation
Possible sepsis	Suspected sepsis in patients who present with altered mental state, low blood pressure (Systolic less than 100) or raised respiratory rate (rate more than 22). In children, age specific physiological tools should be used to determine if possibly septic
History of head injury	A history of a recent physically traumatic event involving the head. Usually this will be reported by the patient, but if the patient has been unconscious, this history should be sought from a reliable witness
Persistent vomiting	Vomiting that is continuous or that occurs without any respite between episodes
Inappropriate history	When the history (story) given does not explain the physical findings, it is termed inappropriate. This is important as it is a marker of safeguarding concerns in both adults and children
Auricular haematoma	A tense haematoma (usually post traumatic) in the outer ear
Vertigo	An acute feeling of spinning or dizziness, possibly accompanied by nausea and vomiting
Recent hearing loss	Loss of hearing in one or both ears within the previous week

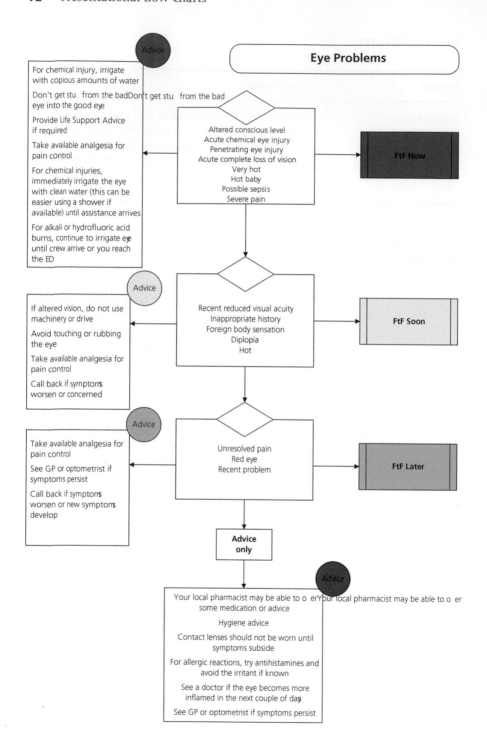

Advice

Eye Problems

For chemical injury, irrigate with copious amounts of water

Don't get stu from the badDon't get stu from the bad eye into the good eye

Provide Life Support Advice if required

Take available analgesia for pain control

For chemical injuries, immediately irrigate the eye with clean water (this can be easier using a shower if available) until assistance arrives

For alkali or hydrofluoric acid burns, continue to irrigate eye until crew arrive or you reach the ED

Altered conscious level
Acute chemical eye injury
Penetrating eye injury
Acute complete loss of vision
Very hot
Hot baby
Possible sepsis
Severe pain

FtF Now

Advice

If altered vision, do not use machinery or drive

Avoid touching or rubbing the eye

Take available analgesia for pain control

Call back if symptoms worsen or concerned

Recent reduced visual acuity
Inappropriate history
Foreign body sensation
Diplopia
Hot

FtF Soon

Advice

Take available analgesia for pain control

See GP or optometrist if symptoms persist

Call back if symptoms worsen or new symptoms develop

Unresolved pain
Red eye
Recent problem

FtF Later

Advice only

Advice

Your local pharmacist may be able to o erYour local pharmacist may be able to o er some medication or advice

Hygiene advice

Contact lenses should not be worn until symptoms subside

For allergic reactions, try antihistamines and avoid the irritant if known

See a doctor if the eye becomes more inflamed in the next couple of days

See GP or optometrist if symptoms persist

Eye problems

See also	Chart notes
Facial problems	This is a presentation-defined flow diagram designed to allow accurate prioritisation of patients attending with conditions affecting the eye. A number of specific discriminators have been used including *Acute Chemical injury*, which indicates that immediate action is required, *Penetrating eye injury* and *Acute complete loss of vision*

Specific discriminators	Explanation
Acute chemical eye injury	Any substance splashed into or placed into the eye within the past 12 hours that caused stinging, burning or reduced vision should be assumed to have caused chemical injury
Penetrating eye injury	A recent physically traumatic event involving penetration of the globe
Acute complete loss of vision	Loss of vision in one or both eyes within the preceding 24 hours which has not returned to normal
Possible sepsis	Suspected sepsis in patients who present with altered mental state, low blood pressure (Systolic less than 100) or raised respiratory rate (rate more than 22). In children, age specific physiological tools should be used to determine if possibly septic
Recent reduced visual acuity	Any reduction in corrected visual acuity within the past 7 days
Inappropriate history	When the history (story) given does not explain the physical findings, it is termed inappropriate. This is important as it is a marker of safeguarding concerns in both adults and children
Foreign body sensation	A sensation of something in the eye, often expressed as scraping or grittiness
Diplopia	Double vision which resolves when one eye is closed
Red eye	Any redness to the eye. A red eye may be painful or painless and may be complete or partial

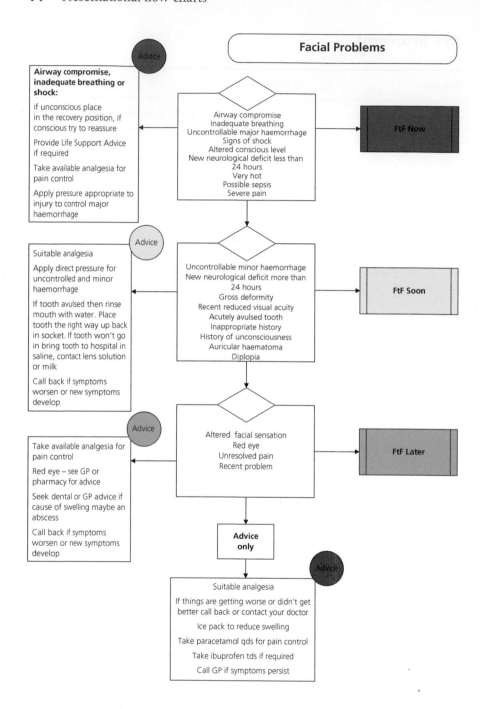

Facial Problems

Airway compromise, inadequate breathing or shock:

if unconscious place in the recovery position, if conscious try to reassure

Provide Life Support Advice if required

Take available analgesia for pain control

Apply pressure appropriate to injury to control major haemorrhage

Advice

Airway compromise
Inadequate breathing
Uncontrollable major haemorrhage
Signs of shock
Altered conscious level
New neurological deficit less than 24 hours
Very hot
Possible sepsis
Severe pain

FtF Now

Advice

Suitable analgesia

Apply direct pressure for uncontrolled and minor haemorrhage

If tooth avulsed then rinse mouth with water. Place tooth the right way up back in socket. If tooth won't go in bring tooth to hospital in saline, contact lens solution or milk

Call back if symptoms worsen or new symptoms develop

Uncontrollable minor haemorrhage
New neurological deficit more than 24 hours
Gross deformity
Recent reduced visual acuity
Acutely avulsed tooth
Inappropriate history
History of unconsciousness
Auricular haematoma
Diplopia

FtF Soon

Advice

Take available analgesia for pain control

Red eye – see GP or pharmacy for advice

Seek dental or GP advice if cause of swelling maybe an abscess

Call back if symptoms worsen or new symptoms develop

Altered facial sensation
Red eye
Unresolved pain
Recent problem

FtF Later

Advice only

Advice

Suitable analgesia

If things are getting worse or didn't get better call back or contact your doctor

Ice pack to reduce swelling

Take paracetamol qds for pain control

Take ibuprofen tds if required

Call GP if symptoms persist

Facial problems

See also	Chart notes
Dental problems Ear problems Eye problems Head injury	This presentation-defined flow diagram has been designed to allow accurate prioritisation of patients presenting with problems affecting the face. A number of general discriminators have been used including *Life Threat*, *Haemorrhage* and *Pain*

Specific discriminators	Explanation
New neurological deficit less than 24 hours	Any loss of neurological function that has come on within the previous 24 hours. This might include altered or lost sensation, weakness of the limbs (either transiently or permanently) and alterations in bladder or bowel function
Possible sepsis	Suspected sepsis in patients who present with altered mental state, low blood pressure (Systolic less than 100) or raised respiratory rate (rate more than 22). In children, age specific physiological tools should be used to determine if possibly septic
New neurological deficit more than 24 hours	Any loss of neurological function including altered or lost sensation, weakness of the limbs (either transiently or permanently) and alterations in bladder or bowel function
Gross deformity	This will always be subjective. Gross and abnormal angulation or rotation is implied
Recent reduced visual acuity	Any reduction in corrected visual acuity within the past 7 days
Acutely avulsed tooth	A tooth that has been avulsed intact within the previous 24 hours
Inappropriate history	When the history (story) given does not explain the physical findings, it is termed inappropriate. This is important as it is a marker of safeguarding concerns in both adults and children
Auricular haematoma	A tense haematoma (usually post traumatic) in the outer ear
Diplopia	Double vision which resolves when one eye is closed
Altered facial sensation	Any alteration of sensation on the face
Red eye	Any redness to the eye. A red eye may be painful or painless and may be complete or partial

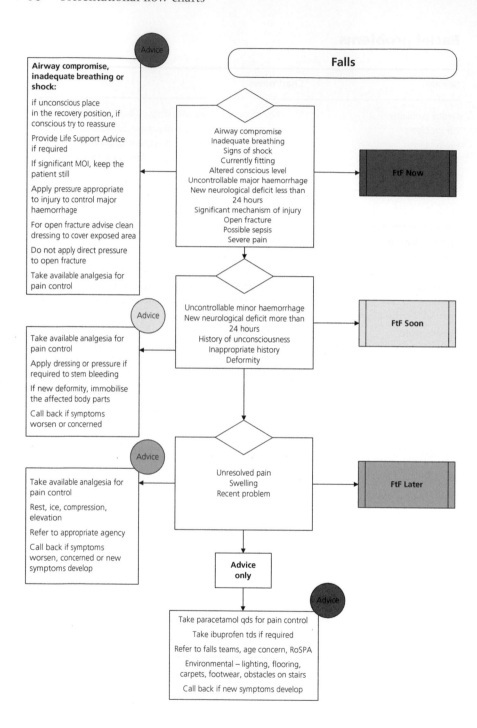

Falls

Airway compromise, inadequate breathing or shock:

if unconscious place in the recovery position, if conscious try to reassure

Provide Life Support Advice if required

If significant MOI, keep the patient still

Apply pressure appropriate to injury to control major haemorrhage

For open fracture advise clean dressing to cover exposed area

Do not apply direct pressure to open fracture

Take available analgesia for pain control

Airway compromise
Inadequate breathing
Signs of shock
Currently fitting
Altered conscious level
Uncontrollable major haemorrhage
New neurological deficit less than 24 hours
Significant mechanism of injury
Open fracture
Possible sepsis
Severe pain

FtF Now

Take available analgesia for pain control

Apply dressing or pressure if required to stem bleeding

If new deformity, immobilise the affected body parts

Call back if symptoms worsen or concerned

Uncontrollable minor haemorrhage
New neurological deficit more than 24 hours
History of unconsciousness
Inappropriate history
Deformity

FtF Soon

Take available analgesia for pain control

Rest, ice, compression, elevation

Refer to appropriate agency

Call back if symptoms worsen, concerned or new symptoms develop

Unresolved pain
Swelling
Recent problem

FtF Later

Advice only

Take paracetamol qds for pain control

Take ibuprofen tds if required

Refer to falls teams, age concern, RoSPA

Environmental – lighting, flooring, carpets, footwear, obstacles on stairs

Call back if new symptoms develop

Falls

See also	Chart notes
Collapsed adult	This is a presentation-defined flow diagram. Many patients who present with a history of falls have suffered trauma as a result, and their priority will reflect the injuries suffered. Some, however, may have had a serious underlying pathology which has caused them to fall or may have developed complications after falling. This chart is designed to allow accurate prioritisation whether the injury or underlying cause is more pressing. A number of general discriminators have been included to ensure that patients suffering from serious underlying conditions or limb-threatening injuries are given a high priority

Specific discriminators	Explanation
New neurological deficit less than 24 hours	Any loss of neurological function that has come on within the previous 24 hours. This might include altered or lost sensation, weakness of the limbs (either transiently or permanently) and alterations in bladder or bowel function
Significant mechanism of injury	Penetrating injuries (stab or gunshot) and injuries with high energy transfer
Open fracture	All wounds in the vicinity of a fracture should be regarded with suspicion. If there is any possibility of communication between the wound and the fracture, then the fracture should be assumed to be open
Possible sepsis	Suspected sepsis in patients who present with altered mental state, low blood pressure (Systolic less than 100) or raised respiratory rate (rate more than 22). In children, age specific physiological tools should be used to determine if possibly septic
New neurological deficit more than 24 hours	Any loss of neurological function including altered or lost sensation, weakness of the limbs (either transiently or permanently) and alterations in bladder or bowel function
Inappropriate history	When the history (story) given does not explain the physical findings, it is termed inappropriate. This is important as it is a marker of safeguarding concerns in both adults and children
Deformity	This will always be subjective. Abnormal angulation or rotation is implied
Swelling	An abnormal increase in size

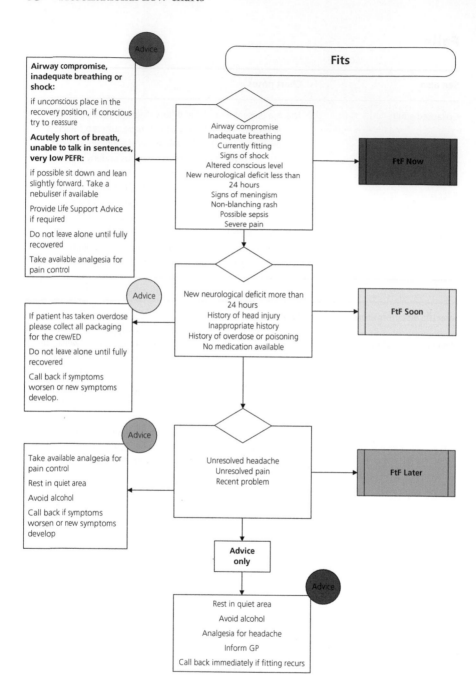

Fits

Advice

Airway compromise, inadequate breathing or shock:

if unconscious place in the recovery position, if conscious try to reassure

Acutely short of breath, unable to talk in sentences, very low PEFR:

if possible sit down and lean slightly forward. Take a nebuliser if available

Provide Life Support Advice if required

Do not leave alone until fully recovered

Take available analgesia for pain control

Airway compromise
Inadequate breathing
Currently fitting
Signs of shock
Altered conscious level
New neurological deficit less than 24 hours
Signs of meningism
Non-blanching rash
Possible sepsis
Severe pain

FtF Now

Advice

If patient has taken overdose please collect all packaging for the crew/ED

Do not leave alone until fully recovered

Call back if symptoms worsen or new symptoms develop.

New neurological deficit more than 24 hours
History of head injury
Inappropriate history
History of overdose or poisoning
No medication available

FtF Soon

Advice

Take available analgesia for pain control

Rest in quiet area

Avoid alcohol

Call back if symptoms worsen or new symptoms develop

Unresolved headache
Unresolved pain
Recent problem

FtF Later

Advice only

Advice

Rest in quiet area
Avoid alcohol
Analgesia for headache
Inform GP
Call back immediately if fitting recurs

Fits

See also	Chart notes
Head injury Headache Overdose and poisoning	This is a presentation-defined flow diagram. The chart is designed to allow rapid categorisation of patients who are currently fitting or who have fitted. A number of general discriminators are used including *Life Threat*, *Conscious Level* and *Temperature*. Specific discriminators include *Signs of meningism* and a focal or progressive loss of function

Specific discriminators	Explanation
Currently fitting	Patients who are in the tonic or clonic stages of a grand mal convulsion and patients currently experiencing partial fits fulfil this criterion
New neurological deficit less than 24 hours	Any loss of neurological function that has come on within the previous 24 hours. This might include altered or lost sensation, weakness of the limbs (either transiently or permanently) and alterations in bladder or bowel function
Signs of meningism	Classically a stiff neck together with headache and photophobia
Non-blanching rash	A rash that does not blanch (go white) when pressure is applied to it. Often tested using a glass tumbler to apply pressure as any colour change can be observed through the bottom of the tumbler
Possible sepsis	Suspected sepsis in patients who present with altered mental state, low blood pressure (Systolic less than 100) or raised respiratory rate (rate more than 22). In children, age specific physiological tools should be used to determine if possibly septic
New neurological deficit more than 24 hours	Any loss of neurological function including altered or lost sensation, weakness of the limbs (either transiently or permanently) and alterations in bladder or bowel function
History of head injury	A history of a recent physically traumatic event involving the head. Usually this will be reported by the patient, but if the patient has been unconscious, this history should be sought from a reliable witness
Inappropriate history	When the history (story) given does not explain the physical findings, it is termed inappropriate. This is important as it is a marker of safeguarding concerns in both adults and children
History of overdose or poisoning	This information may come from others or may be deduced if medication is missing
No medication available	No medication available
Unresolved headache	A headache that has not resolved despite waiting an appropriate time or being given appropriate analgesia

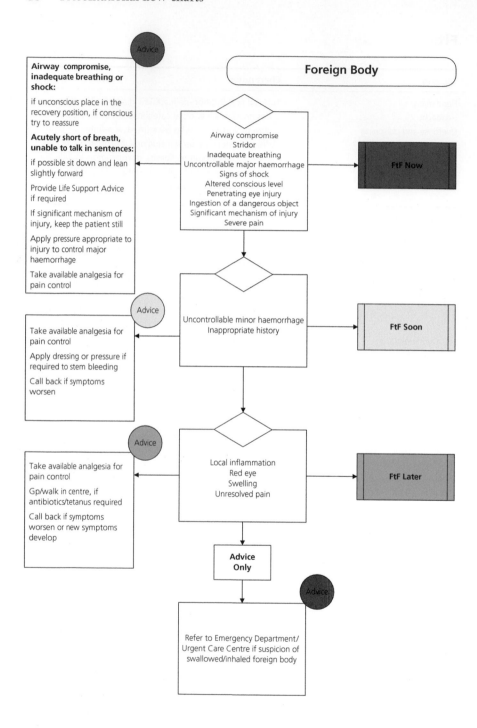

Foreign Body

Advice

Airway compromise, inadequate breathing or shock:

if unconscious place in the recovery position, if conscious try to reassure

Acutely short of breath, unable to talk in sentences:

if possible sit down and lean slightly forward

Provide Life Support Advice if required

If significant mechanism of injury, keep the patient still

Apply pressure appropriate to injury to control major haemorrhage

Take available analgesia for pain control

Airway compromise
Stridor
Inadequate breathing
Uncontrollable major haemorrhage
Signs of shock
Altered conscious level
Penetrating eye injury
Ingestion of a dangerous object
Significant mechanism of injury
Severe pain

FtF Now

Advice

Take available analgesia for pain control

Apply dressing or pressure if required to stem bleeding

Call back if symptoms worsen

Uncontrollable minor haemorrhage
Inappropriate history

FtF Soon

Advice

Take available analgesia for pain control

Gp/walk in centre, if antibiotics/tetanus required

Call back if symptoms worsen or new symptoms develop

Local inflammation
Red eye
Swelling
Unresolved pain

FtF Later

**Advice
Only**

Advice

Refer to Emergency Department/ Urgent Care Centre if suspicion of swallowed/inhaled foreign body

Foreign body

See also	Chart notes
Torso injury Wounds	This is a presentation-defined flow diagram designed to allow accurate prioritisation of patients who present with foreign bodies in any part of their anatomy. The severity of such cases can range from the inconvenient to the life-threatening and this chart is designed to differentiate between these. A number of general discriminators have been used including *Life Threat*, *Haemorrhage* and *Pain*. The only specific discriminator that relates to anatomical site is that of *Penetrating Eye Injury*

Specific discriminators	Explanation
Stridor	This may be an inspiratory or expiratory noise or both. Stridor is heard best on breathing with the mouth open
Penetrating eye injury	A recent physically traumatic event involving penetration of the globe
Ingestion of a dangerous object	Ingestion of a dangerous or potentially dangerous foreign object e.g. button battery, magnets or razor blades which may be a potential threat to life
Significant mechanism of injury	Penetrating injuries (stab or gunshot) and injuries with high energy transfer
Inappropriate history	When the history (story) given does not explain the physical findings, it is termed inappropriate. This is important as it is a marker of safeguarding concerns in both adults and children
Local inflammation	Local inflammation will involve pain, swelling and redness confined to a particular site or area
Red eye	Any redness to the eye. A red eye may be painful or painless and may be complete or partial

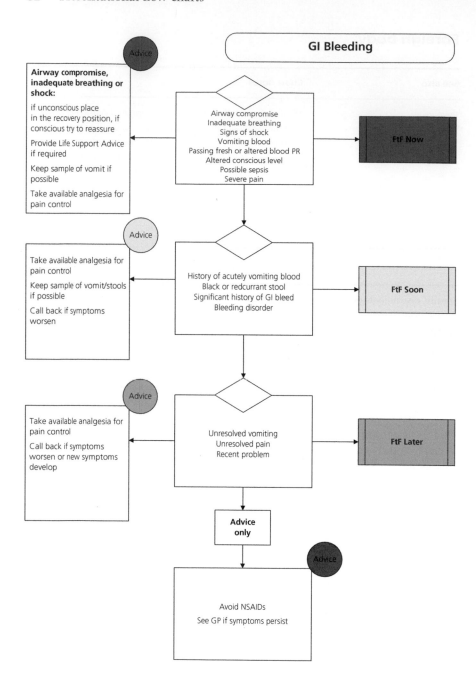

GI Bleeding

Advice

Airway compromise, inadequate breathing or shock:

if unconscious place in the recovery position, if conscious try to reassure

Provide Life Support Advice if required

Keep sample of vomit if possible

Take available analgesia for pain control

Airway compromise
Inadequate breathing
Signs of shock
Vomiting blood
Passing fresh or altered blood PR
Altered conscious level
Possible sepsis
Severe pain

FtF Now

Advice

Take available analgesia for pain control

Keep sample of vomit/stools if possible

Call back if symptoms worsen

History of acutely vomiting blood
Black or redcurrant stool
Significant history of GI bleed
Bleeding disorder

FtF Soon

Advice

Take available analgesia for pain control

Call back if symptoms worsen or new symptoms develop

Unresolved vomiting
Unresolved pain
Recent problem

FtF Later

Advice only

Advice

Avoid NSAIDs
See GP if symptoms persist

GI bleeding

See also	Chart notes
Abdominal pain in adults Abdominal pain in children Diarrhoea and vomiting	This is a presentation-defined flow diagram. Patients may present with GI bleeding either as vomiting fresh or altered blood or by passing blood PR. A number of general discriminators are used including *Life Threat* and *Pain*. Specific discriminators have been selected to indicate the current severity of the GI bleeding. Thus patients vomiting blood or those passing fresh or altered blood PR have a higher category than those with a history of vomiting

Specific discriminators	Explanation
Vomiting blood	Vomited blood may be fresh (bright or dark red) or coffee ground in appearance
Passing fresh or altered blood PR	In active massive GI bleeding, dark red blood will be passed PR. As GI transit time increases, this becomes darker, eventually becoming melaena
Possible sepsis	Suspected sepsis in patients who present with altered mental state, low blood pressure (Systolic less than 100) or raised respiratory rate (rate more than 22). In children, age specific physiological tools should be used to determine if possibly septic
History of acutely vomiting blood	Frank haematemesis, vomiting of altered blood (coffee ground) or of blood mixed in the vomit within the past 24 hours
Black or redcurrant stools	Any blackness fulfils the criteria of black stool while a dark red stool, classically seen in intussusceptions, is redcurrant stool
Significant history of GI bleed	Any history of massive GI bleeding or of any GI bleed associated with oesophageal varices
Bleeding disorder	Congenital or acquired bleeding disorder

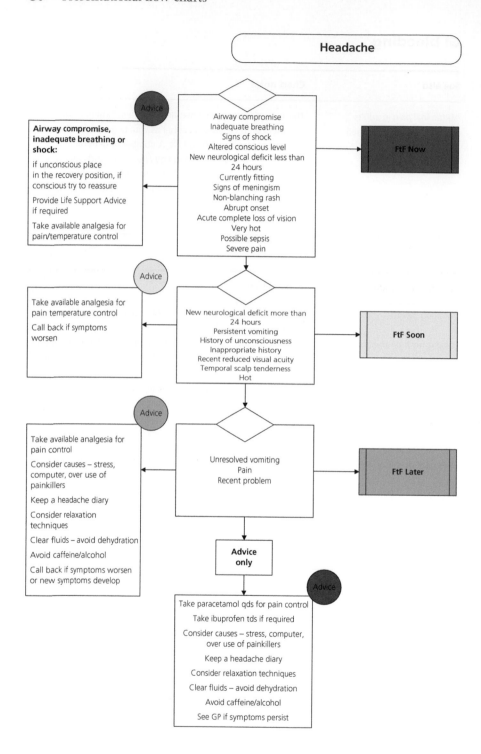

Headache

Airway compromise
Inadequate breathing
Signs of shock
Altered conscious level
New neurological deficit less than
24 hours
Currently fitting
Signs of meningism
Non-blanching rash
Abrupt onset
Acute complete loss of vision
Very hot
Possible sepsis
Severe pain

FtF Now

Advice

Airway compromise, inadequate breathing or shock:

if unconscious place
in the recovery position, if
conscious try to reassure

Provide Life Support Advice
if required

Take available analgesia for
pain/temperature control

Advice

New neurological deficit more than
24 hours
Persistent vomiting
History of unconsciousness
Inappropriate history
Recent reduced visual acuity
Temporal scalp tenderness
Hot

FtF Soon

Take available analgesia for
pain temperature control

Call back if symptoms
worsen

Advice

Unresolved vomiting
Pain
Recent problem

FtF Later

Take available analgesia for
pain control

Consider causes – stress,
computer, over use of
painkillers

Keep a headache diary

Consider relaxation
techniques

Clear fluids – avoid dehydration

Avoid caffeine/alcohol

Call back if symptoms worsen
or new symptoms develop

**Advice
only**

Advice

Take paracetamol qds for pain control

Take ibuprofen tds if required

Consider causes – stress, computer,
over use of painkillers

Keep a headache diary

Consider relaxation techniques

Clear fluids – avoid dehydration

Avoid caffeine/alcohol

See GP if symptoms persist

Headache

See also	Chart notes
Head injury Neck pain	This is a presentation defined-flow diagram. A large number of conditions can present with headache and a number of these require urgent intervention. A number of general discriminators are used including *Life Threat*, *Conscious Level*, *Pain* and *Temperature*. Specific discriminators have been used to identify severe causes such as subarachnoid haemorrhage and meningococcaemia. New neurological signs or symptoms together with reduction in visual acuity and tenderness of the scalp are used to indicate the need for immediate clinical review

Specific discriminators	Explanation
New neurological deficit less than 24 hours	Any loss of neurological function that has come on within the previous 24 hours. This might include altered or lost sensation, weakness of the limbs (either transiently or permanently) and alterations in bladder or bowel function
Signs of meningism	Classically a stiff neck together with headache and photophobia
Non-blanching rash	A rash that does not blanch (go white) when pressure is applied to it. Often tested using a glass tumbler to apply pressure as any colour change can be observed through the bottom of the tumbler
Abrupt onset	Onset within seconds or minutes. May cause waking in sleep
Acute complete loss of vision	Loss of vision in one or both eyes within the preceding 24 hours which has not returned to normal
Possible sepsis	Suspected sepsis in patients who present with altered mental state, low blood pressure (Systolic less than 100) or raised respiratory rate (rate more than 22). In children, age specific physiological tools should be used to determine if possibly septic
New neurological deficit more than 24 hours	Any loss of neurological function including altered or lost sensation, weakness of the limbs (either transiently or permanently) and alterations in bladder or bowel function
Persistent vomiting	Vomiting that is continuous or that occurs without any respite between episodes
Recent reduced visual acuity	Any reduction in corrected visual acuity within the past 7 days
Inappropriate history	When the history (story) given does not explain the physical findings, it is termed inappropriate. This is important as it is a marker of safeguarding concerns in both adults and children
Temporal scalp tenderness	Tenderness on palpation over the temporal area (especially over the artery)
History of unconsciousness	There may be a reliable witness who can state whether the patient was unconscious (and for how long). If not, a patient who is unable to remember the incident should be assumed to have been unconscious

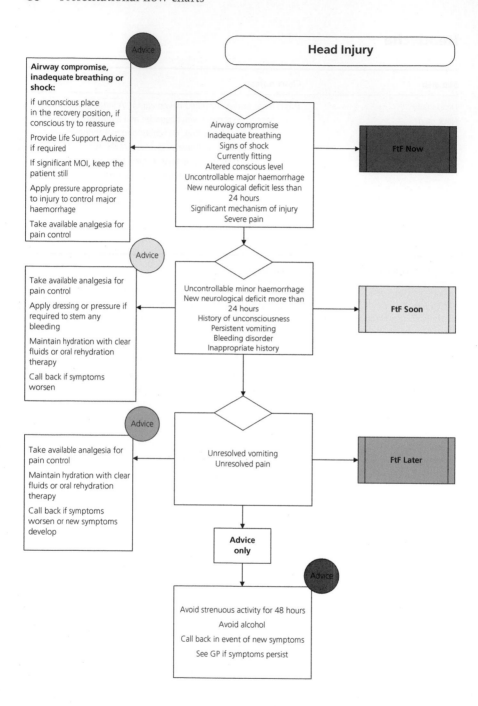

Head Injury

Advice

Airway compromise, inadequate breathing or shock:

if unconscious place in the recovery position, if conscious try to reassure

Provide Life Support Advice if required

If significant MOI, keep the patient still

Apply pressure appropriate to injury to control major haemorrhage

Take available analgesia for pain control

Airway compromise
Inadequate breathing
Signs of shock
Currently fitting
Altered conscious level
Uncontrollable major haemorrhage
New neurological deficit less than 24 hours
Significant mechanism of injury
Severe pain

FtF Now

Advice

Take available analgesia for pain control

Apply dressing or pressure if required to stem any bleeding

Maintain hydration with clear fluids or oral rehydration therapy

Call back if symptoms worsen

Uncontrollable minor haemorrhage
New neurological deficit more than 24 hours
History of unconsciousness
Persistent vomiting
Bleeding disorder
Inappropriate history

FtF Soon

Advice

Take available analgesia for pain control

Maintain hydration with clear fluids or oral rehydration therapy

Call back if symptoms worsen or new symptoms develop

Unresolved vomiting
Unresolved pain

FtF Later

Advice only

Advice

Avoid strenuous activity for 48 hours
Avoid alcohol
Call back in event of new symptoms
See GP if symptoms persist

Head injury

See also	Chart notes
Fits Headache Neck pain	This is a presentation-defined flow diagram. Head injury is an extremely common presentation and its effects may vary from life-threatening extradural haemorrhage to minimal scalp injury. A number of general discriminators have been used including *Life Threat, Conscious Level (both in adults and children), Haemorrhage* and *Pain.* Specific discriminators are included to select those patients with significant mechanism and the development of neurological signs and symptoms, to a higher priority

Specific Discriminators	Explanation
Currently fitting	Patients who are in the tonic or clonic stages of a grand mal convulsion and patients currently experiencing partial fits fulfil this criterion
New neurological deficit less than 24 hours	Any loss of neurological function that has come on within the previous 24 hours. This might include altered or lost sensation, weakness of the limbs (either transiently or permanently) and alterations in bladder or bowel function
Significant mechanism of injury	Penetrating injuries (stab or gunshot) and injuries with high energy transfer
New neurological deficit more than 24 hours	Any loss of neurological function including altered or lost sensation, weakness of the limbs (either transiently or permanently) and alterations in bladder or bowel function
History of unconsciousness	There may be a reliable witness who can state whether the patient was unconscious (and for how long). If not, a patient who is unable to remember the incident should be assumed to have been unconscious
Persistent vomiting	Vomiting that is continuous or that occurs without any respite between episodes
Bleeding disorder	Congenital or acquired bleeding disorder
Inappropriate history	When the history (story) given does not explain the physical findings, it is termed inappropriate. This is important as it is a marker of safeguarding concerns in both adults and children

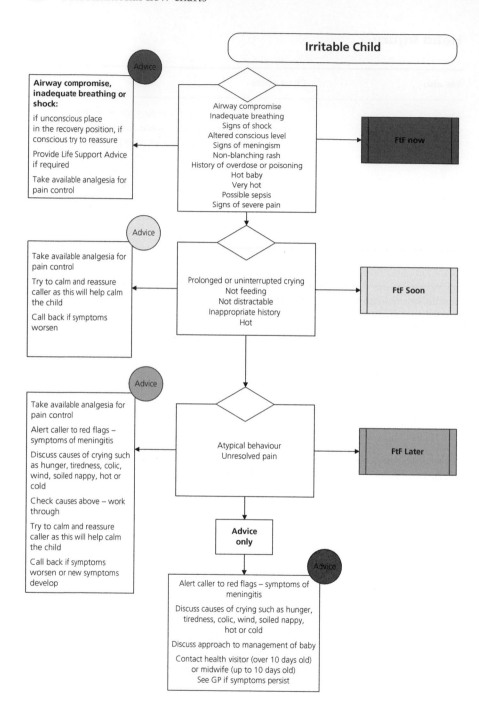

Irritable Child

Airway compromise
Inadequate breathing
Signs of shock
Altered conscious level
Signs of meningism
Non-blanching rash
History of overdose or poisoning
Hot baby
Very hot
Possible sepsis
Signs of severe pain

FtF now

Advice

Airway compromise, inadequate breathing or shock:

if unconscious place in the recovery position, if conscious try to reassure

Provide Life Support Advice if required

Take available analgesia for pain control

Prolonged or uninterrupted crying
Not feeding
Not distractable
Inappropriate history
Hot

FtF Soon

Advice

Take available analgesia for pain control

Try to calm and reassure caller as this will help calm the child

Call back if symptoms worsen

Atypical behaviour
Unresolved pain

FtF Later

Advice

Take available analgesia for pain control

Alert caller to red flags – symptoms of meningitis

Discuss causes of crying such as hunger, tiredness, colic, wind, soiled nappy, hot or cold

Check causes above – work through

Try to calm and reassure caller as this will help calm the child

Call back if symptoms worsen or new symptoms develop

Advice only

Advice

Alert caller to red flags – symptoms of meningitis

Discuss causes of crying such as hunger, tiredness, colic, wind, soiled nappy, hot or cold

Discuss approach to management of baby

Contact health visitor (over 10 days old) or midwife (up to 10 days old)
See GP if symptoms persist

Irritable child

See also	Chart notes
Crying baby Unwell child Unwell newborn Worried parent	This is a presentation-defined flow diagram. It is designed to be used in **children over the age of 12 months**. A number of general discriminators have been used including *Life Threat*, *Conscious Level* and *Pain*. Specific discriminators include those which allow recognition of more specific pathologies such as septicaemia or which indicate that a more serious pathology might exist. If the patient is under 28 days, the Unwell newborn chart should be used

Specific discriminators	Explanation
Signs of meningism	Classically a stiff neck together with headache and photophobia
Non-blanching rash	A rash that does not blanch (go white) when pressure is applied to it. Often tested using a glass tumbler to apply pressure as any colour change can be observed through the bottom of the tumbler
History of overdose or poisoning	This information may come from others or may be deduced if medication is missing
Signs of severe pain	Young children and babies in severe pain cannot complain. They will usually cry out continuously and inconsolably and be tachycardic. They may well exhibit signs such as pallor and sweating
Possible sepsis	Suspected sepsis in patients who present with altered mental state, low blood pressure (Systolic less than 100) or raised respiratory rate (rate more than 22). In children, age specific physiological tools should be used to determine if possibly septic
Prolonged or uninterrupted crying	A child who has cried continuously for 2 hours or more fulfils this criterion
Not feeding	Children who do not take any solid or liquid (as appropriate) by mouth. Children who take the food but always vomit afterwards may also fulfil this criterion
Not distractible	Children who are distressed by pain or other things who cannot be distracted by conversation or play fulfil this criterion
Inappropriate history	When the history (story) given does not explain the physical findings, it is termed inappropriate. This is important as it is a marker of safeguarding concerns in both adults and children
Atypical behaviour	Children who behave in a way that is not usual in the given situation. The carers will often volunteer this information. Such children are often referred to as fractious or 'out of sorts'

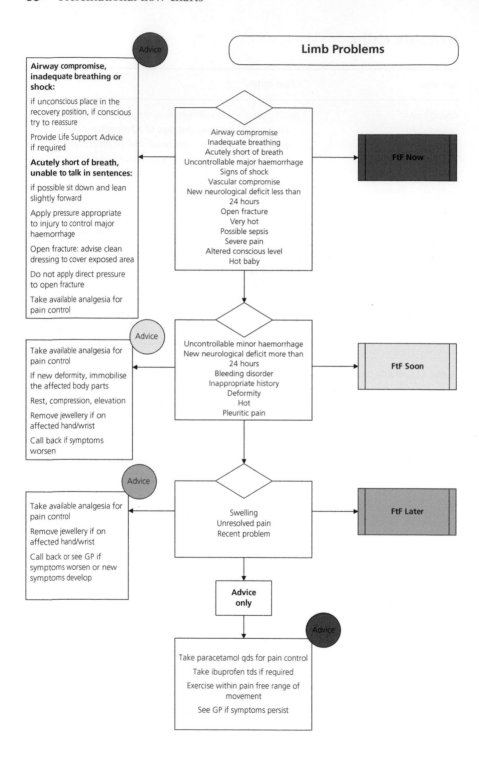

Limb Problems

Airway compromise, inadequate breathing or shock:

if unconscious place in the recovery position, if conscious try to reassure

Provide Life Support Advice if required

Acutely short of breath, unable to talk in sentences:

if possible sit down and lean slightly forward

Apply pressure appropriate to injury to control major haemorrhage

Open fracture: advise clean dressing to cover exposed area

Do not apply direct pressure to open fracture

Take available analgesia for pain control

Advice

Airway compromise
Inadequate breathing
Acutely short of breath
Uncontrollable major haemorrhage
Signs of shock
Vascular compromise
New neurological deficit less than 24 hours
Open fracture
Very hot
Possible sepsis
Severe pain
Altered conscious level
Hot baby

FtF Now

Advice

Take available analgesia for pain control

If new deformity, immobilise the affected body parts

Rest, compression, elevation

Remove jewellery if on affected hand/wrist

Call back if symptoms worsen

Uncontrollable minor haemorrhage
New neurological deficit more than 24 hours
Bleeding disorder
Inappropriate history
Deformity
Hot
Pleuritic pain

FtF Soon

Advice

Take available analgesia for pain control

Remove jewellery if on affected hand/wrist

Call back or see GP if symptoms worsen or new symptoms develop

Swelling
Unresolved pain
Recent problem

FtF Later

Advice only

Advice

Take paracetamol qds for pain control

Take ibuprofen tds if required

Exercise within pain free range of movement

See GP if symptoms persist

Limb problems

See also	Chart notes
Limping child	This is a presentation-defined flow diagram. Injuries to the limbs, while rarely life-threatening, may cause considerable morbidity. A number of general discriminators are used including *Life Threat*, *Haemorrhage* and *Pain*. Specific discriminators are included to ensure that limb-threatening injuries are seen and treated urgently. Discriminators are also included to remind the triage practitioner to consider the signs and symptoms of thromboembolic disease and its complications

Specific discriminators	Explanation
Acutely short of breath	Shortness of breath that comes on suddenly or a sudden exacerbation of chronic shortness of breath
Vascular compromise	There will be a combination of pallor, coldness, altered sensation and pain with or without absent pulses distal to the injury
New neurological deficit less than 24 hours	Any loss of neurological function that has come on within the previous 24 hours. This might include altered or lost sensation, weakness of the limbs (either transiently or permanently) and alterations in bladder or bowel function
Open fracture	All wounds in the vicinity of a fracture should be regarded with suspicion. If there is any possibility of communication between the wound and the fracture, then the fracture should be assumed to be open
Possible sepsis	Suspected sepsis in patients who present with altered mental state, low blood pressure (Systolic less than 100) or raised respiratory rate (rate more than 22). In children, age specific physiological tools should be used to determine if possibly septic
New neurological deficit more than 24 hours	Any loss of neurological function including altered or lost sensation, weakness of the limbs (either transiently or permanently) and alterations in bladder or bowel function
Bleeding disorder	Congenital or acquired bleeding disorder
Inappropriate history	When the history (story) given does not explain the physical findings, it is termed inappropriate. This is important as it is a marker of safeguarding concerns in both adults and children
Deformity	This will always be subjective. Abnormal angulation or rotation is implied
Pleuritic pain	A sharp, localised pain in the chest that worsens on breathing, coughing or sneezing
Swelling	An abnormal increase in size

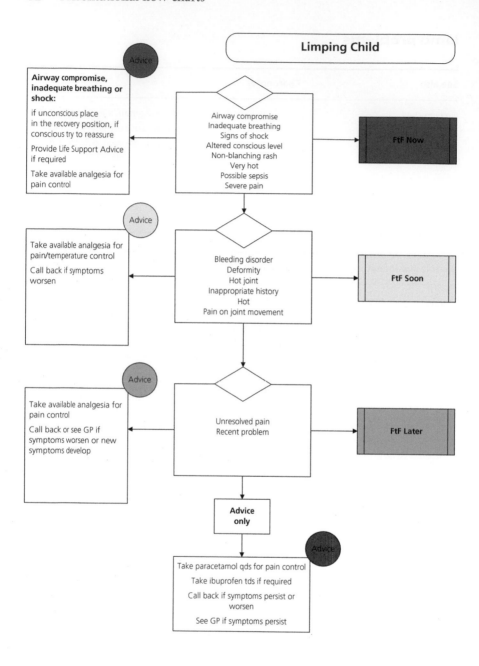

Limping Child

Advice

Airway compromise, inadequate breathing or shock:

if unconscious place in the recovery position, if conscious try to reassure

Provide Life Support Advice if required

Take available analgesia for pain control

Airway compromise
Inadequate breathing
Signs of shock
Altered conscious level
Non-blanching rash
Very hot
Possible sepsis
Severe pain

FtF Now

Advice

Take available analgesia for pain/temperature control

Call back if symptoms worsen

Bleeding disorder
Deformity
Hot joint
Inappropriate history
Hot
Pain on joint movement

FtF Soon

Advice

Take available analgesia for pain control

Call back or see GP if symptoms worsen or new symptoms develop

Unresolved pain
Recent problem

FtF Later

Advice only

Advice

Take paracetamol qds for pain control

Take ibuprofen tds if required

Call back if symptoms persist or worsen

See GP if symptoms persist

Limping child

	Chart notes
Limb injuries	This is a presentation-defined flow diagram. Children who present with limp range from those who have suffered a minor soft tissue injury to the foot or ankle to those who have developed septic arthritis of the hip. This chart is designed to allow accurate prioritisation of such children. A number of general discriminators are used including *Life Threat*, *Pain* and *Temperature*. Specific discriminators have been included to allow children with more urgent pathologies which threaten distal function from being accurately identified and those in whom the limp is a sinister sign of systemic disease from being spotted quickly

Specific discriminators	Explanation
Non-blanching rash	A rash that does not blanch (go white) when pressure is applied to it. Often tested using a glass tumbler to apply pressure as any colour change can be observed through the bottom of the tumbler
Possible sepsis	Suspected sepsis in patients who present with altered mental state, low blood pressure (Systolic less than 100) or raised respiratory rate (rate more than 22). In children, age specific physiological tools should be used to determine if possibly septic
Bleeding disorder	Congenital or acquired bleeding disorder
Deformity	This will always be subjective. Abnormal angulation or rotation is implied
Inappropriate history	When the history (story) given does not explain the physical findings, it is termed inappropriate. This is important as it is a marker of safeguarding concerns in both adults and children
Hot joint	Any warmth around a joint fulfils this criterion. Often accompanied by redness
Pain on joint movement	This can be pain on either active (patient) movement or passive (examiner) movement

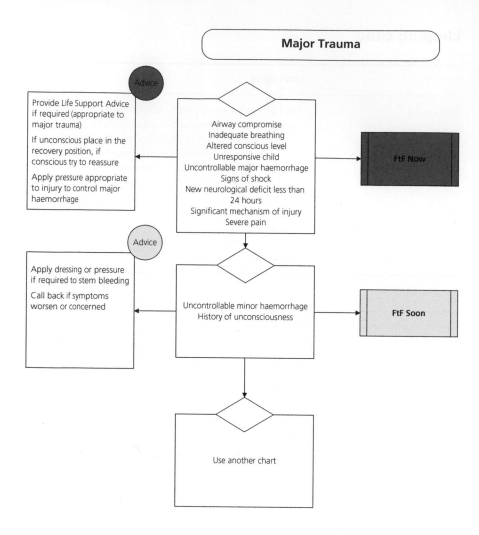

Major Trauma

Advice

Provide Life Support Advice
if required (appropriate to
major trauma)

If unconscious place in the
recovery position, if
conscious try to reassure

Apply pressure appropriate
to injury to control major
haemorrhage

Airway compromise
Inadequate breathing
Altered conscious level
Unresponsive child
Uncontrollable major haemorrhage
Signs of shock
New neurological deficit less than
24 hours
Significant mechanism of injury
Severe pain

FtF Now

Advice

Apply dressing or pressure
if required to stem bleeding

Call back if symptoms
worsen or concerned

Uncontrollable minor haemorrhage
History of unconsciousness

FtF Soon

Use another chart

Major trauma

See also	Chart notes
	Most health care providers know what is implied by major trauma, but it is a strange presentation in that it is defined not by the patients or their injury but on some judgement of that injury by carers at the scene or triage practitioner. For this reason, it is impossible to categorise a patient with this presentation as less than 'face to face Soon'. If it is necessary to do this, then a deliberate decision needs to be made that the original description of the patient as having suffered major trauma was incorrect, and the patient should be categorised using a different presentational flow diagram
	A number of general discriminators have been used including *Life Threat*, *Haemorrhage*, *Conscious Level* and *Pain*. Specific discriminators are designed to ensure that patients with a significant mechanism of injury are given immediate care

Specific discriminators	Explanation
New neurological deficit less than 24 hours	Any loss of neurological function that has come on within the previous 24 hours. This might include altered or lost sensation, weakness of the limbs (either transiently or permanently) and alterations in bladder or bowel function
Significant mechanism of injury	Penetrating injuries (stab or gunshot) and injuries with high energy transfer
History of unconsciousness	There may be a reliable witness who can state whether the patient was unconscious (and for how long). If not, a patient who is unable to remember the incident should be assumed to have been unconscious

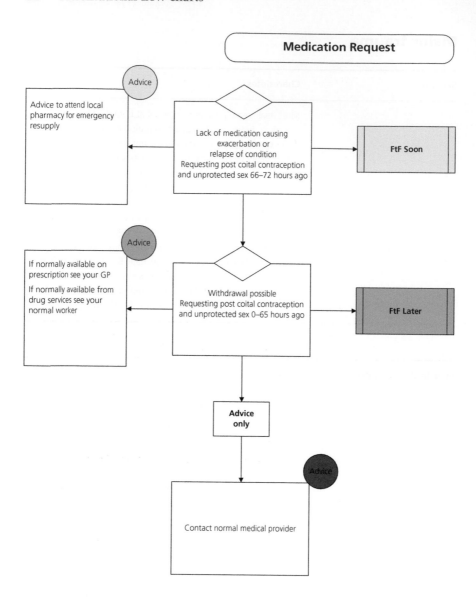

Medication request

	Chart notes
	This is presentation-defined flow diagram designed to prioritise those who request medications. It is impossible to categorise a patient with this presentation as 'face to face Now'. If the patient has general discriminators which suggest a 'face to face Now' categorisation or a 'face to face Soon' categorisation, then another chart should be used. For that reason there are no general discriminators in this chart

Specific discriminators	Explanation
Lack of medication causing exacerbation or relapse of condition	Lack of regular medications such as insulin which may cause exacerbation or relapse of condition if not obtained soon
Requesting post-coital contraception and unprotected sex 66–72 hours ago	There is a window of opportunity for post-coital contraception which best evidence suggests ends at 72 hours
Withdrawal possible	Where the lack of medication will lead to symptoms of drug/substance withdrawal or other unwanted effects
Requesting post-coital contraception and unprotected sex 0–65 hours ago	Medication is required but there is a larger window of opportunity for obtaining it

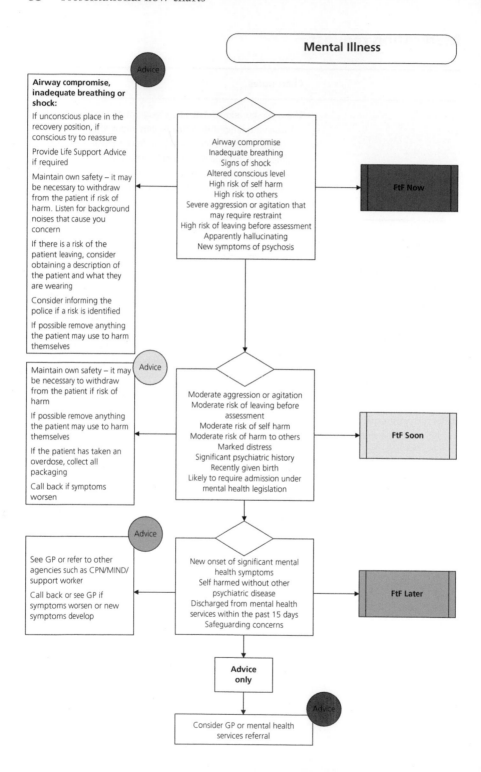

Mental Illness

Advice

Airway compromise, inadequate breathing or shock:

If unconscious place in the recovery position, if conscious try to reassure

Provide Life Support Advice if required

Maintain own safety – it may be necessary to withdraw from the patient if risk of harm. Listen for background noises that cause you concern

If there is a risk of the patient leaving, consider obtaining a description of the patient and what they are wearing

Consider informing the police if a risk is identified

If possible remove anything the patient may use to harm themselves

Airway compromise
Inadequate breathing
Signs of shock
Altered conscious level
High risk of self harm
High risk to others
Severe aggression or agitation that may require restraint
High risk of leaving before assessment
Apparently hallucinating
New symptoms of psychosis

FtF Now

Advice

Maintain own safety – it may be necessary to withdraw from the patient if risk of harm

If possible remove anything the patient may use to harm themselves

If the patient has taken an overdose, collect all packaging

Call back if symptoms worsen

Moderate aggression or agitation
Moderate risk of leaving before assessment
Moderate risk of self harm
Moderate risk of harm to others
Marked distress
Significant psychiatric history
Recently given birth
Likely to require admission under mental health legislation

FtF Soon

Advice

See GP or refer to other agencies such as CPN/MIND/support worker

Call back or see GP if symptoms worsen or new symptoms develop

New onset of significant mental health symptoms
Self harmed without other psychiatric disease
Discharged from mental health services within the past 15 days
Safeguarding concerns

FtF Later

Advice only

Advice

Consider GP or mental health services referral

Mental illness

See also	Chart notes
Apparently drunk Behaving strangely	This is a presentation-defined flow diagram which has been designed to allow clinical prioritisation of patients who present with known or newly declared mental illness. A number of general discriminators have been used including *Life Threat* and *Conscious Level*. This chart is designed to allow assessment of both physical and psychiatric aspects of the presentation Specific discriminators are included to allow accurate prioritisation of patients with a known significant psychiatric history and those who have a degree of risk of causing harm to others or to themselves. Patients who suffer from marked distress are placed in 'face to face Soon' category

Specific discriminators	Explanation
High risk of self harm	An initial view of the risk of harm to self can be formed by considering the patient's behaviour. Patients who are threatening to harm themselves and who are actively seeking the means to do so are at high risk
High risk to others	An initial view of the risk of harm to others can be judged by assessing posture (tense, clenched), speech (loud, using threatening words) loud background noise can be an indicator and motor behaviour (restless, pacing, lunging at others). High risk should be assumed if weapons and potential victims are available and no controls are already in place
Severe aggression or agitation that may require restraint	Aggression and agitation of such a degree that restraint may be required at short notice to manage the risk of harm to self or others
Marked distress	Patients who are markedly physically or emotionally upset fulfil this criterion
Significant psychiatric history	A history of a major psychiatric illness or event
Likely to require admission under mental health legislation	Patients with significant psychiatric symptoms who are likely to require admission under mental health legislation

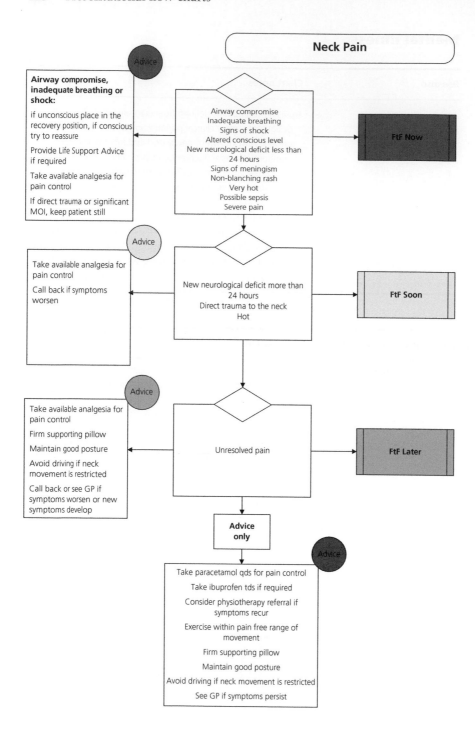

Neck Pain

Advice

Airway compromise, inadequate breathing or shock:

if unconscious place in the recovery position, if conscious try to reassure

Provide Life Support Advice if required

Take available analgesia for pain control

If direct trauma or significant MOI, keep patient still

Airway compromise
Inadequate breathing
Signs of shock
Altered conscious level
New neurological deficit less than 24 hours
Signs of meningism
Non-blanching rash
Very hot
Possible sepsis
Severe pain

FtF Now

Advice

Take available analgesia for pain control

Call back if symptoms worsen

New neurological deficit more than 24 hours
Direct trauma to the neck
Hot

FtF Soon

Advice

Take available analgesia for pain control

Firm supporting pillow

Maintain good posture

Avoid driving if neck movement is restricted

Call back or see GP if symptoms worsen or new symptoms develop

Unresolved pain

FtF Later

Advice only

Advice

Take paracetamol qds for pain control

Take ibuprofen tds if required

Consider physiotherapy referral if symptoms recur

Exercise within pain free range of movement

Firm supporting pillow

Maintain good posture

Avoid driving if neck movement is restricted

See GP if symptoms persist

Neck pain

See also	Chart notes
Back pain Headache	This is a presentation-defined flow diagram. Pain in the neck may arise because of local pathology or meningeal irritation. This chart is designed to allow rapid identification of patients presented with symptoms or signs which indicate more urgent pathologies. A number of general discriminators are used including *Life Threat*, *Pain* and *Temperature*. The specific discriminators which indicate meningitis are included under 'face to face Now' category

Specific discriminators	Explanation
New neurological deficit less than 24 hrs	Any loss of neurological function that has come on within the previous 24 hours. This might include altered or lost sensation, weakness of the limbs (either transiently or permanently) and alterations in bladder or bowel function
Signs of meningism	Classically a stiff neck together with headache and photophobia
Non-blanching rash	A rash that does not blanch (go white) when pressure is applied to it. Often tested using a glass tumbler to apply pressure as any colour change can be observed through the bottom of the tumbler
Possible sepsis	Suspected sepsis in patients who present with altered mental state, low blood pressure (Systolic less than 100) or raised respiratory rate (rate more than 22). In children, age specific physiological tools should be used to determine if possibly septic
New neurological deficit more than 24 hours	Any loss of neurological function including altered or lost sensation, weakness of the limbs (either transiently or permanently) and alterations in bladder or bowel function
Direct trauma to the neck	This may be top to bottom (loading) for instance when something falls on the head, bending (forwards, backwards or to the side), twisting or distracting such as in hanging

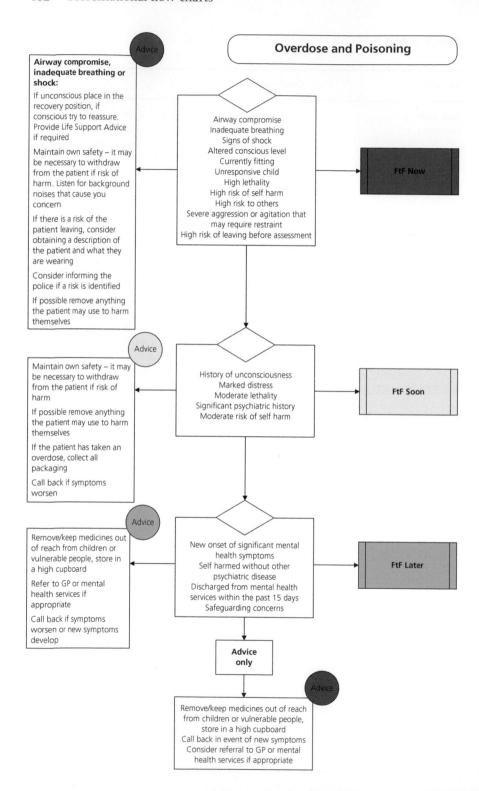

Overdose and Poisoning

Advice

Airway compromise, inadequate breathing or shock:

If unconscious place in the recovery position, if conscious try to reassure. Provide Life Support Advice if required

Maintain own safety – it may be necessary to withdraw from the patient if risk of harm. Listen for background noises that cause you concern

If there is a risk of the patient leaving, consider obtaining a description of the patient and what they are wearing

Consider informing the police if a risk is identified

If possible remove anything the patient may use to harm themselves

Airway compromise
Inadequate breathing
Signs of shock
Altered conscious level
Currently fitting
Unresponsive child
High lethality
High risk of self harm
High risk to others
Severe aggression or agitation that may require restraint
High risk of leaving before assessment

FtF Now

Advice

Maintain own safety – it may be necessary to withdraw from the patient if risk of harm

If possible remove anything the patient may use to harm themselves

If the patient has taken an overdose, collect all packaging

Call back if symptoms worsen

History of unconsciousness
Marked distress
Moderate lethality
Significant psychiatric history
Moderate risk of self harm

FtF Soon

Advice

Remove/keep medicines out of reach from children or vulnerable people, store in a high cupboard

Refer to GP or mental health services if appropriate

Call back if symptoms worsen or new symptoms develop

New onset of significant mental health symptoms
Self harmed without other psychiatric disease
Discharged from mental health services within the past 15 days
Safeguarding concerns

FtF Later

Advice only

Advice

Remove/keep medicines out of reach from children or vulnerable people, store in a high cupboard
Call back in event of new symptoms
Consider referral to GP or mental health services if appropriate

Overdose and poisoning

See also	Chart notes
Self-harm	This is a presentation-defined flow diagram. The flow chart has been designed to allow both the physical and psychiatric aspects of overdose to be considered and to ensure accurate prioritisation of patients from both perspectives. It also allows prioritisation of patients who have been accidentally (or deliberately) poisoned
	A number of general discriminators have been used including *Life Threat* and *Unconscious Level*. Specific discriminators include the assessed lethality of the overdose (which can be decided following discussion with a Poisons Centre) and an assessment of the risk of further attempts at self-harm

Specific discriminators	Explanation
High lethality	Lethality is the potential of the substance taken to cause harm. Advice from a Poisons Centre may be required to establish the level of risk of serious illness or death. If in doubt, assume a high risk
High risk of self harm	An initial view of the risk of harm to self can be formed by considering the patient's behaviour. Patients who are threatening to harm themselves and who are actively seeking the means to do so are at high risk
High risk of leaving before assessment	Active, credible threats to leave prior to assessment pose a high risk
History of unconsciousness	There may be a reliable witness who can state whether the patient was unconscious (and for how long). If not, a patient who is unable to remember the incident should be assumed to have been unconscious
Marked distress	Patients who are markedly physically or emotionally upset fulfil this criterion
Moderate lethality	Lethality is the potential of the substance taken to cause serious illness or death. Advice from a Poisons Centre may be required to establish the level of risk to the patient
Significant psychiatric history	A history of a major psychiatric illness or event
Self harmed without other psychiatric disease	Patients who have harmed themselves (for the first or subsequent time) who do not have a mental health diagnosis

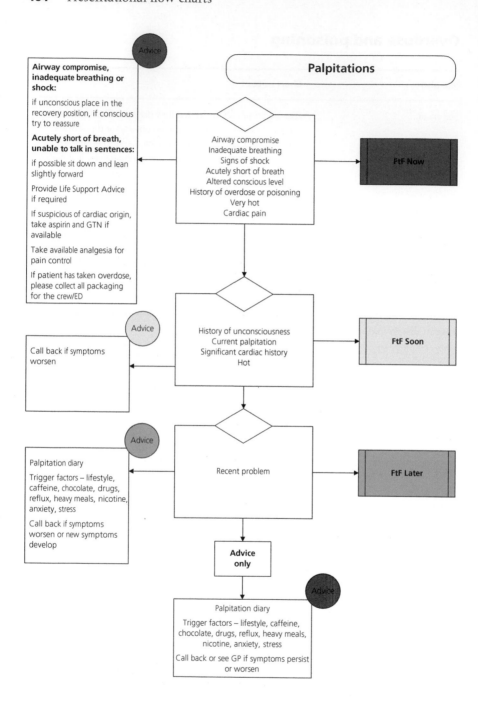

Palpitations

Advice

Airway compromise, inadequate breathing or shock:

if unconscious place in the recovery position, if conscious try to reassure

Acutely short of breath, unable to talk in sentences:

if possible sit down and lean slightly forward

Provide Life Support Advice if required

If suspicious of cardiac origin, take aspirin and GTN if available

Take available analgesia for pain control

If patient has taken overdose, please collect all packaging for the crew/ED

Airway compromise
Inadequate breathing
Signs of shock
Acutely short of breath
Altered conscious level
History of overdose or poisoning
Very hot
Cardiac pain

FtF Now

Advice

Call back if symptoms worsen

History of unconsciousness
Current palpitation
Significant cardiac history
Hot

FtF Soon

Advice

Palpitation diary

Trigger factors – lifestyle, caffeine, chocolate, drugs, reflux, heavy meals, nicotine, anxiety, stress

Call back if symptoms worsen or new symptoms develop

Recent problem

FtF Later

Advice only

Advice

Palpitation diary

Trigger factors – lifestyle, caffeine, chocolate, drugs, reflux, heavy meals, nicotine, anxiety, stress

Call back or see GP if symptoms persist or worsen

Palpitations

See also	Chart notes
Chest pain Collapsed adult Unwell adult	This is a presentation-defined flow diagram designed to allow the accurate prioritisation of those patients that present with a chief complaint of palpitations. Palpitations can have many causes ranging from the effects of ischaemic heart disease and other cardiac abnormalities to anxiety. Whatever the cause, it is their effect on circulation and their propensity to develop into life-threatening dysrhythmias that determine the clinical priority of the patient. Thus this chart is written to ensure that the signs and symptoms of cardiac insufficiency are included in the 'face to face Now' category, together with historical pointers to potential early problems

Specific discriminators	Explanation
Acutely short of breath	Shortness of breath that comes on suddenly or a sudden exacerbation of chronic shortness of breath
History of overdose or poisoning	This information may come from others or may be deduced if medication is missing
Cardiac pain	Classically a severe dull 'gripping' or 'heavy' pain in the centre of the chest, radiating to the left arm or to the neck. May be associated with sweating and nausea
History of unconsciousness	There may be a reliable witness who can state whether the patient was unconscious (and for how long). If not, a patient who is unable to remember the incident should be assumed to have been unconscious
Current palpitation	A feeling of the heart racing (often described as a fluttering) that is still present
Significant cardiac history	A known recurrent dysrhythmia which has life-threatening effects is significant, as is a known cardiac condition that may deteriorate rapidly

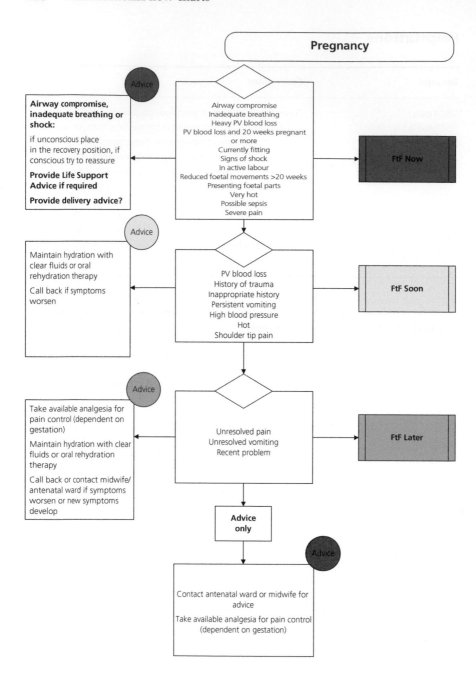

Pregnancy

Airway compromise, inadequate breathing or shock:

if unconscious place in the recovery position, if conscious try to reassure

Provide Life Support Advice if required

Provide delivery advice?

Advice

Airway compromise
Inadequate breathing
Heavy PV blood loss
PV blood loss and 20 weeks pregnant or more
Currently fitting
Signs of shock
In active labour
Reduced foetal movements >20 weeks
Presenting foetal parts
Very hot
Possible sepsis
Severe pain

FtF Now

Advice

Maintain hydration with clear fluids or oral rehydration therapy

Call back if symptoms worsen

PV blood loss
History of trauma
Inappropriate history
Persistent vomiting
High blood pressure
Hot
Shoulder tip pain

FtF Soon

Advice

Take available analgesia for pain control (dependent on gestation)

Maintain hydration with clear fluids or oral rehydration therapy

Call back or contact midwife/antenatal ward if symptoms worsen or new symptoms develop

Unresolved pain
Unresolved vomiting
Recent problem

FtF Later

Advice only

Advice

Contact antenatal ward or midwife for advice

Take available analgesia for pain control (dependent on gestation)

Pregnancy

See also	Chart notes
PV bleeding	This is a presentation-defined flow diagram. Pregnant women may access Emergency care at all stages of pregnancy and with a variety of complaints. Some may be unaware of their pregnancy. A number of general discriminators have been used including *Pain* and *Conscious Level*. Specific discriminators are designed to allow early recognition of complications of pregnancy at all stages

Specific discriminators	Explanation
Heavy PV blood loss	PV loss is extremely difficult to assess. The presence of large clots or constant flow fulfils this criterion. The use of a large number of sanitary towels is suggestive of heavy loss
PV blood loss and 20 weeks pregnant or more	Any loss of blood per vaginum in a woman known to be beyond the 20th week of pregnancy
In active labour	A woman who has regular and frequent painful contractions fulfils this criterion
Reduced foetal movements >20 weeks	Absent or reduced foetal movements during the previous 12 hours in a woman known to be beyond the 20th week of pregnancy
Presenting foetal parts	Crowning or presentation of any other foetal part in the vagina
Possible sepsis	Suspected sepsis in patients who present with altered mental state, low blood pressure (Systolic less than 100) or raised respiratory rate (rate more than 22). In children, age specific physiological tools should be used to determine if possibly septic
PV blood loss	Any loss of blood PV
History of trauma	A history of a recent physically traumatic event
Inappropriate history	When the history (story) given does not explain the physical findings, it is termed inappropriate. This is important as it is a marker of safeguarding concerns in both adults and children
High blood pressure	A history of raised blood pressure or a raised blood pressure on examination
Shoulder tip pain	Pain felt in the tip of the shoulder. This often indicates diaphragmatic irritation

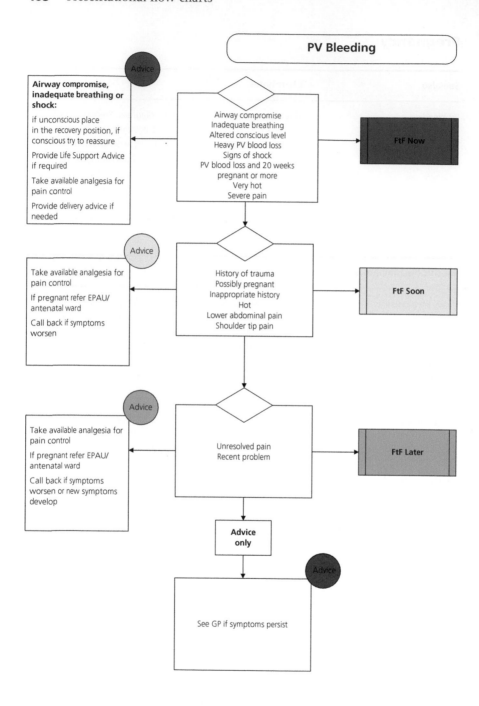

PV Bleeding

Advice

Airway compromise, inadequate breathing or shock:

if unconscious place in the recovery position, if conscious try to reassure

Provide Life Support Advice if required

Take available analgesia for pain control

Provide delivery advice if needed

Airway compromise
Inadequate breathing
Altered conscious level
Heavy PV blood loss
Signs of shock
PV blood loss and 20 weeks pregnant or more
Very hot
Severe pain

FtF Now

Advice

Take available analgesia for pain control

If pregnant refer EPAU/ antenatal ward

Call back if symptoms worsen

History of trauma
Possibly pregnant
Inappropriate history
Hot
Lower abdominal pain
Shoulder tip pain

FtF Soon

Advice

Take available analgesia for pain control

If pregnant refer EPAU/ antenatal ward

Call back if symptoms worsen or new symptoms develop

Unresolved pain
Recent problem

FtF Later

Advice only

Advice

See GP if symptoms persist

PV bleeding

See also	Chart notes
Lower abdominal pain Pregnancy	This is a presentation-defined flow diagram. PV bleeding may occur in pregnant and non-pregnant women and may have a large number of undefined causes. A number of general discriminators are used including *Life Threat*, *Haemorrhage* and *Pain*.

Specific discriminators	Explanation
Heavy PV blood loss	PV loss is extremely difficult to assess. The presence of large clots or constant flow fulfils this criterion. The use of a large number of sanitary towels is suggestive of heavy loss
PV blood loss and 20 weeks pregnant or more	Any loss of blood PV in a woman known to be beyond the 20th week of pregnancy
Possibly pregnant	Any woman whose normal menstruation has failed to occur is possibly pregnant. Furthermore, any woman of childbearing age who has unprotected sex should be considered to be potentially pregnant
Inappropriate history	When the history (story) given does not explain the physical findings, it is termed inappropriate. This is important as it is a marker of safeguarding concerns in both adults and children
Lower abdominal pain	Any pain felt in the abdomen; association with PV bleeding may indicate ectopic pregnancy or miscarriage
Shoulder tip pain	Pain felt in the tip of the shoulder. This often indicates diaphragmatic irritation

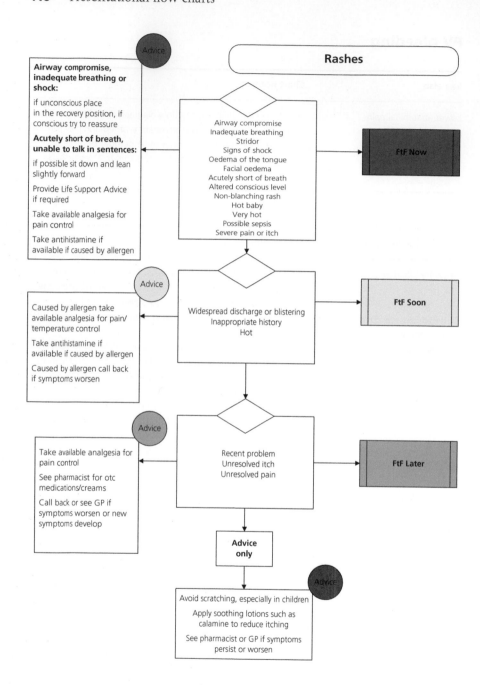

Rashes

Advice

Airway compromise, inadequate breathing or shock:

if unconscious place in the recovery position, if conscious try to reassure

Acutely short of breath, unable to talk in sentences:

if possible sit down and lean slightly forward

Provide Life Support Advice if required

Take available analgesia for pain control

Take antihistamine if available if caused by allergen

Airway compromise
Inadequate breathing
Stridor
Signs of shock
Oedema of the tongue
Facial oedema
Acutely short of breath
Altered conscious level
Non-blanching rash
Hot baby
Very hot
Possible sepsis
Severe pain or itch

FtF Now

Advice

Caused by allergen take available analgesia for pain/ temperature control

Take antihistamine if available if caused by allergen

Caused by allergen call back if symptoms worsen

Widespread discharge or blistering
Inappropriate history
Hot

FtF Soon

Advice

Take available analgesia for pain control

See pharmacist for otc medications/creams

Call back or see GP if symptoms worsen or new symptoms develop

Recent problem
Unresolved itch
Unresolved pain

FtF Later

Advice only

Advice

Avoid scratching, especially in children

Apply soothing lotions such as calamine to reduce itching

See pharmacist or GP if symptoms persist or worsen

Rashes

See also	Chart notes
Allergy Bites and stings Unwell adult Unwell child	This is a presentation-defined flow diagram. A rash may signify serious disease such as meningococcal septicaemia or may be a sign of a chronic non-acute problem such as psoriasis. Two general discriminators – *Life Threat* and *Temperature* – are used in this chart. A larger number of specific discriminators are included in the 'face to face Now' and 'face to face Soon' categories to ensure that more *serious* conditions are suitably triaged. In particular, non-blanching rash and associations of acute anaphylaxis appear at the 'face to face Now' level

Specific discriminators	Explanation
Stridor	This may be an inspiratory or expiratory noise or both. Stridor is heard best on breathing with the mouth open
Oedema of the tongue	Swelling of the tongue of any degree
Facial oedema	Diffuse swelling around the face usually involving the lips
Acutely short of breath	Shortness of breath that comes on suddenly or a sudden exacerbation of chronic shortness of breath
Non-blanching rash	A rash that does not blanch (go white) when pressure is applied to it. Often tested using a glass tumbler to apply pressure as any colour change can be observed through the bottom of the tumbler
Possible sepsis	Suspected sepsis in patients who present with altered mental state, low blood pressure (Systolic less than 100) or raised respiratory rate (rate more than 22). In children, age specific physiological tools should be used to determine if possibly septic
Widespread discharge or blistering	Any discharging or blistering eruption covering more than 10% body surface area
Inappropriate history	When the history (story) given does not explain the physical findings, it is termed inappropriate. This is important as it is a marker of safeguarding concerns in both adults and children

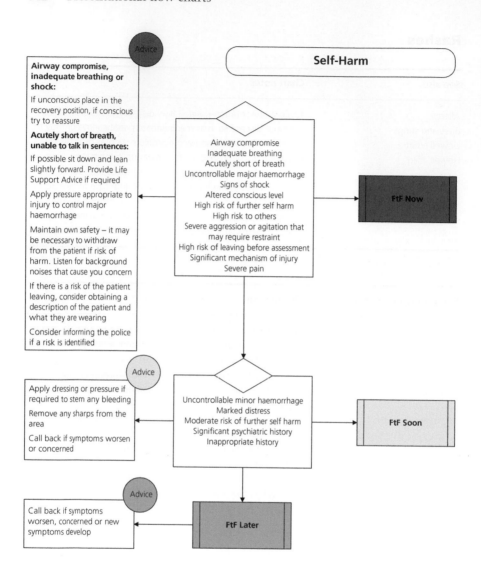

Self-Harm

Advice

Airway compromise, inadequate breathing or shock:

If unconscious place in the recovery position, if conscious try to reassure

Acutely short of breath, unable to talk in sentences:

If possible sit down and lean slightly forward. Provide Life Support Advice if required

Apply pressure appropriate to injury to control major haemorrhage

Maintain own safety – it may be necessary to withdraw from the patient if risk of harm. Listen for background noises that cause you concern

If there is a risk of the patient leaving, consider obtaining a description of the patient and what they are wearing

Consider informing the police if a risk is identified

Airway compromise
Inadequate breathing
Acutely short of breath
Uncontrollable major haemorrhage
Signs of shock
Altered conscious level
High risk of further self harm
High risk to others
Severe aggression or agitation that may require restraint
High risk of leaving before assessment
Significant mechanism of injury
Severe pain

FtF Now

Advice

Apply dressing or pressure if required to stem any bleeding

Remove any sharps from the area

Call back if symptoms worsen or concerned

Uncontrollable minor haemorrhage
Marked distress
Moderate risk of further self harm
Significant psychiatric history
Inappropriate history

FtF Soon

Advice

Call back if symptoms worsen, concerned or new symptoms develop

FtF Later

Self-harm

See also	Chart notes
Overdose and poisoning Mental illness	This is a presentation-defined flow diagram. This flow diagram has been designed to allow accurate prioritisation of patients who have caused physical harm to themselves. This chart is designed to allow assessment of both physical and psychiatric aspects of the presentation A number of general discriminators are used including *Life Threat*, *Haemorrhage*, *Conscious Level* and *Pain*. Specific discriminators are included to allow accurate prioritisation of patients with the significant mechanism of injury and those who have risk of further self-harm.

Specific discriminators	Explanation
Acutely short of breath	Shortness of breath that comes on suddenly or a sudden exacerbation of chronic shortness of breath
High risk of further self harm	An initial view of the risk of harm to self can be formed by considering the patient's behaviour. Patients who are threatening to harm themselves and who are actively seeking the means to do so are at high risk
High risk to others	An initial view of the risk of harm to others can be judged by assessing posture (tense, clenched), speech (loud, using threatening words) loud background noise can be an indicator and motor behaviour (restless, pacing, lunging at others). High risk should be assumed if weapons and potential victims are available and no controls are already in place
Significant mechanism of injury	Penetrating injuries (stab or gunshot) and injuries with high energy transfer
Marked distress	Patients who are markedly physically or emotionally upset fulfil this criterion
Moderate risk of further self harm	An initial view of the risk of harm to self can be formed by considering the patient's behaviour. Patients without a significant history of self harm, who are not actively trying to harm themselves, but who profess the desire to harm themselves are at moderate risk
Significant psychiatric history	A history of a major psychiatric illness or event
Inappropriate history	When the history (story) given does not explain the physical findings, it is termed inappropriate. This is important as it is a marker of safeguarding concerns in both adults and children

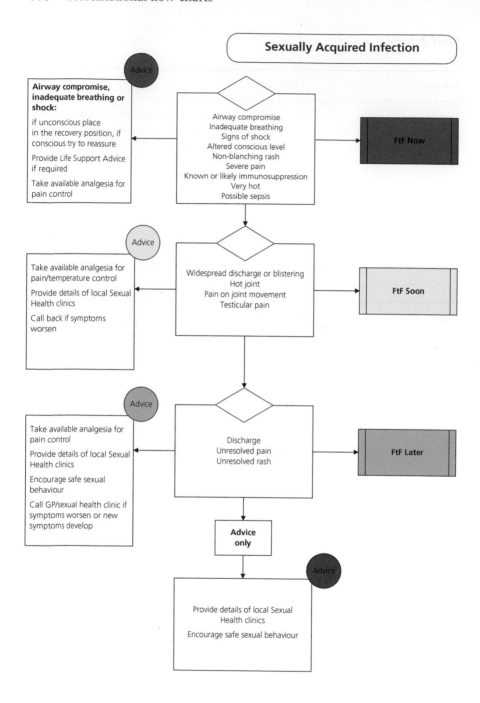

Sexually Acquired Infection

Advice

Airway compromise, inadequate breathing or shock:

if unconscious place in the recovery position, if conscious try to reassure

Provide Life Support Advice if required

Take available analgesia for pain control

Airway compromise
Inadequate breathing
Signs of shock
Altered conscious level
Non-blanching rash
Severe pain
Known or likely immunosuppression
Very hot
Possible sepsis

FtF Now

Advice

Take available analgesia for pain/temperature control

Provide details of local Sexual Health clinics

Call back if symptoms worsen

Widespread discharge or blistering
Hot joint
Pain on joint movement
Testicular pain

FtF Soon

Advice

Take available analgesia for pain control

Provide details of local Sexual Health clinics

Encourage safe sexual behaviour

Call GP/sexual health clinic if symptoms worsen or new symptoms develop

Discharge
Unresolved pain
Unresolved rash

FtF Later

Advice only

Advice

Provide details of local Sexual Health clinics

Encourage safe sexual behaviour

Sexually-acquired infection

	Chart notes
	This is a presentation-defined flow diagram which has been included to allow prioritisation of patients who present with known or obvious sexually acquired infection. A number of general discriminators are used including *Life Threat*, *Pain* and *Temperature*. Specific discriminators have been added to allow identification of more urgent conditions such as gonococcaemia It is important to ensure that preconceptions about disposal of these patients do not prevent appropriate triage

Specific discriminators	Explanation
Non-blanching rash	A rash that does not blanch (go white) when pressure is applied to it. Often tested using a glass tumbler to apply pressure as any colour change can be observed through the bottom of the tumbler
Known or likely immunosuppression	Any patient who is known or likely to be immunosuppressed including those on immunosuppressive drugs (including long-term steroids)
Possible sepsis	Suspected sepsis in patients who present with altered mental state, low blood pressure (Systolic less than 100) or raised respiratory rate (rate more than 22). In children, age specific physiological tools should be used to determine if possibly septic
Widespread discharge or blistering	Any discharging or blistering eruption covering more than 10% body surface area
Hot joint	Any warmth around a joint fulfils this criterion. Often accompanied by redness
Pain on joint movement	This can be pain on either active (patient) movement or passive (examiner) movement
Testicular pain	Pain in the testicles
Discharge	In the context of sexually-acquired infection, this is any discharge from the penis or abnormal discharge from the vagina

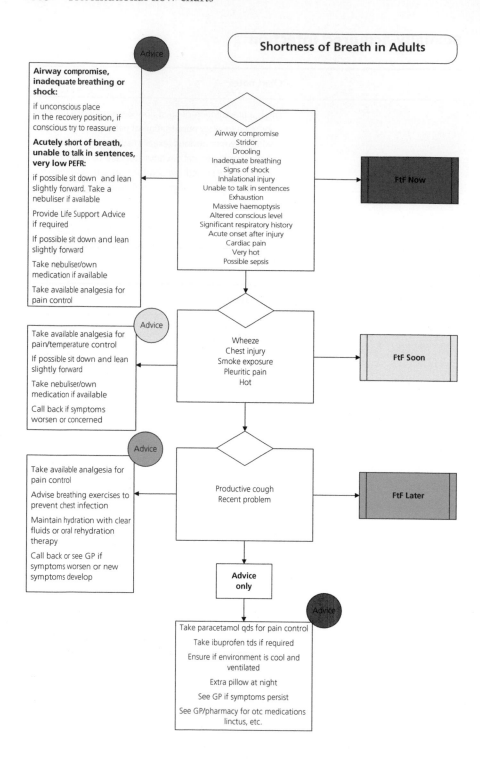

Shortness of Breath in Adults

Airway compromise, inadequate breathing or shock:

if unconscious place in the recovery position, if conscious try to reassure

Acutely short of breath, unable to talk in sentences, very low PEFR:

if possible sit down and lean slightly forward. Take a nebuliser if available

Provide Life Support Advice if required

If possible sit down and lean slightly forward

Take nebuliser/own medication if available

Take available analgesia for pain control

Advice

Airway compromise
Stridor
Drooling
Inadequate breathing
Signs of shock
Inhalational injury
Unable to talk in sentences
Exhaustion
Massive haemoptysis
Altered conscious level
Significant respiratory history
Acute onset after injury
Cardiac pain
Very hot
Possible sepsis

FtF Now

Take available analgesia for pain/temperature control

If possible sit down and lean slightly forward

Take nebuliser/own medication if available

Call back if symptoms worsen or concerned

Advice

Wheeze
Chest injury
Smoke exposure
Pleuritic pain
Hot

FtF Soon

Take available analgesia for pain control

Advise breathing exercises to prevent chest infection

Maintain hydration with clear fluids or oral rehydration therapy

Call back or see GP if symptoms worsen or new symptoms develop

Advice

Productive cough
Recent problem

FtF Later

Advice only

Advice

Take paracetamol qds for pain control

Take ibuprofen tds if required

Ensure if environment is cool and ventilated

Extra pillow at night

See GP if symptoms persist

See GP/pharmacy for otc medications linctus, etc.

Shortness of breath in adults

See also	Chart notes
Asthma Shortness of breath in children Unwell adult	This is a presentation-defined flow diagram. Shortness of breath may be the presenting symptom for a number of cardiovascular and respiratory problems. A number of general discriminators are used including *Life Threat* and *Temperature*. Specific discriminators include those which are present in severe asthma, chronic obstructive pulmonary disease and ischaemic heart disease

Specific discriminators	Explanation
Stridor	This may be an inspiratory or expiratory noise or both. Stridor is heard best on breathing with the mouth open
Drooling	Saliva running from the mouth as a result of being unable to swallow
Inhalational injury	A history of being confined in a smoke filled space is the most reliable indicator of smoke inhalation. Carbon deposits around the mouth and nose and hoarse voice may be present. History is also the most reliable way of diagnosing inhalation of chemicals – there will not necessarily be any signs
Unable to talk in sentences	Patients who are so breathless that they cannot complete relatively short sentences in one breath
Exhaustion	Exhausted patients appear to reduce the effort they make to breathe despite continuing respiratory insufficiency. This is preterminal
Massive haemoptysis	Coughing up large amounts of fresh or clotted blood. Not to be confused with streaks of blood in saliva
Significant respiratory history	A history of previous life-threatening episodes of a respiratory condition (e.g. COPD) is significant as is brittle asthma
Acute onset after injury	Onset of symptoms immediately within 24 hours of a physically traumatic event
Cardiac pain	Classically a severe dull 'gripping' or 'heavy' pain in the centre of the chest, radiating to the left arm or to the neck. May be associated with sweating and nausea
Possible sepsis	Suspected sepsis in patients who present with altered mental state, low blood pressure (Systolic less than 100) or raised respiratory rate (rate more than 22). In children, age specific physiological tools should be used to determine if possibly septic
Wheeze	This can be audible wheeze or a feeling of wheeze. Very severe airway obstruction is silent (no air can move)
Chest injury	Any injury to the area below the clavicles and above the level of the lowest rib. Injury to the lower part of the chest can cause underlying damage to abdominal organs
Smoke exposure	Smoke inhalation should be assumed if the patient has been confined in a smoke-filled space. Physical signs such as oral or nasal soot are less reliable but significant if present
Pleuritic pain	A sharp, localised pain in the chest that worsens on breathing, coughing or sneezing
Productive cough	A cough which is productive of phlegm, whatever the colour

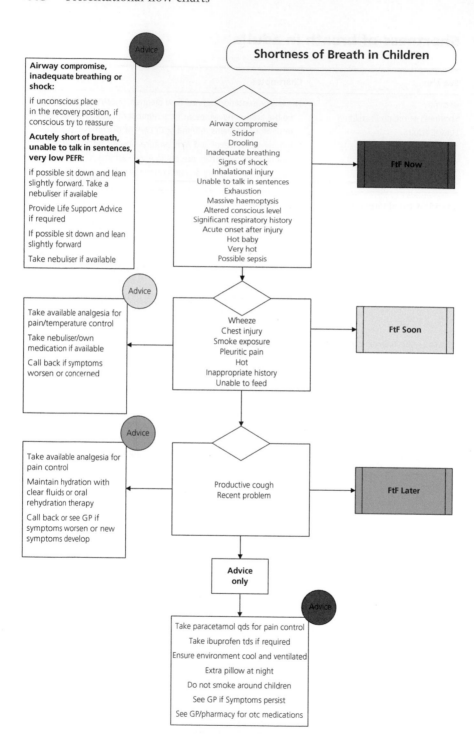

Advice

Shortness of Breath in Children

Airway compromise, inadequate breathing or shock:

if unconscious place in the recovery position, if conscious try to reassure

Acutely short of breath, unable to talk in sentences, very low PEFR:

if possible sit down and lean slightly forward. Take a nebuliser if available

Provide Life Support Advice if required

If possible sit down and lean slightly forward

Take nebuliser if available

Airway compromise
Stridor
Drooling
Inadequate breathing
Signs of shock
Inhalational injury
Unable to talk in sentences
Exhaustion
Massive haemoptysis
Altered conscious level
Significant respiratory history
Acute onset after injury
Hot baby
Very hot
Possible sepsis

FtF Now

Advice

Take available analgesia for pain/temperature control

Take nebuliser/own medication if available

Call back if symptoms worsen or concerned

Wheeze
Chest injury
Smoke exposure
Pleuritic pain
Hot
Inappropriate history
Unable to feed

FtF Soon

Advice

Take available analgesia for pain control

Maintain hydration with clear fluids or oral rehydration therapy

Call back or see GP if symptoms worsen or new symptoms develop

Productive cough
Recent problem

FtF Later

Advice only

Advice

Take paracetamol qds for pain control
Take ibuprofen tds if required
Ensure environment cool and ventilated
Extra pillow at night
Do not smoke around children
See GP if Symptoms persist
See GP/pharmacy for otc medications

Shortness of breath in children

See also	Chart notes
Asthma Unwell child Unwell newborn	This is a presentation-defined flow diagram which applies to children. A number of general discriminators are used including *Life Threat* and *Temperature*. Specific discriminators have been included to allow accurate identification of children who suffer from the severe effects of asthma and those in whom there is more serious pathology. If the patient is under 28 days, the Unwell newborn chart should be used

Specific discriminators	Explanation
Stridor	This may be an inspiratory or expiratory noise or both. Stridor is heard best on breathing with the mouth open
Drooling	Saliva running from the mouth as a result of being unable to swallow
Inhalational injury	A history of being confined in a smoke filled space is the most reliable indicator of smoke inhalation. Carbon deposits around the mouth and nose and hoarse voice may be present. History is also the most reliable way of diagnosing inhalation of chemicals – there will not necessarily be any signs
Unable to talk in sentences	Patients who are so breathless that they cannot complete relatively short sentences in one breath
Exhaustion	Exhausted patients appear to reduce the effort they make to breathe despite continuing respiratory insufficiency. This is pre-terminal
Significant respiratory history	A history of previous life-threatening episodes of a respiratory condition (e.g. COPD) is significant as is brittle asthma
Acute onset after injury	Onset of symptoms immediately within 24 hours of a physically traumatic event
Possible sepsis	Suspected sepsis in patients who present with altered mental state, low blood pressure (Systolic less than 100) or raised respiratory rate (rate more than 22). In children, age specific physiological tools should be used to determine if possibly septic
Massive haemoptysis	Coughing up large amounts of fresh or clotted blood. Not to be confused with streaks of blood in saliva
Wheeze	This can be audible wheeze or a feeling of wheeze. Very severe airway obstruction is silent (no air can move)
Chest injury	Any injury to the area below the clavicles and above the level of the lowest rib. Injury to the lower part of the chest can cause underlying damage to abdominal organs
Smoke exposure	Smoke inhalation should be assumed if the patient has been confined in a smoke-filled space. Physical signs such as oral or nasal soot are less reliable but significant if present
Pleuritic pain	A sharp, localised pain in the chest that worsens on breathing, coughing or sneezing
Inappropriate history	When the history (story) given does not explain the physical findings, it is termed inappropriate. This is important as it is a marker of safeguarding concerns in both adults and children
Unable to feed	This is usually reported by the parents. Children who will not take any solid or liquid (as appropriate) by mouth
Productive cough	A cough which is productive of phlegm, whatever the colour

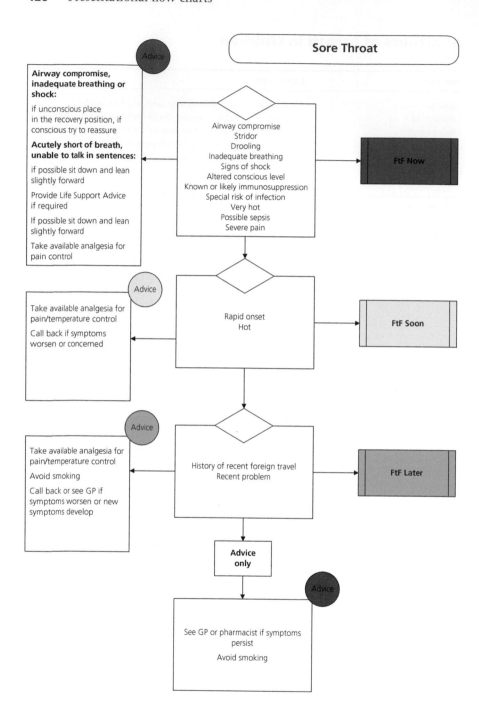

Sore Throat

Advice

Airway compromise, inadequate breathing or shock:

if unconscious place in the recovery position, if conscious try to reassure

Acutely short of breath, unable to talk in sentences:

if possible sit down and lean slightly forward

Provide Life Support Advice if required

If possible sit down and lean slightly forward

Take available analgesia for pain control

Airway compromise
Stridor
Drooling
Inadequate breathing
Signs of shock
Altered conscious level
Known or likely immunosuppression
Special risk of infection
Very hot
Possible sepsis
Severe pain

FtF Now

Advice

Take available analgesia for pain/temperature control

Call back if symptoms worsen or concerned

Rapid onset
Hot

FtF Soon

Advice

Take available analgesia for pain/temperature control

Avoid smoking

Call back or see GP if symptoms worsen or new symptoms develop

History of recent foreign travel
Recent problem

FtF Later

Advice only

Advice

See GP or pharmacist if symptoms persist

Avoid smoking

Sore throat

See also	Chart notes
Shortness of breath in adults Shortness of breath in children Unwell adult Unwell child Unwell newborn	This is a presentation-defined flow diagram designed to allow accurate prioritisation for patients presenting with sore throat. As problems with the throat can affect the airway, there are a number of conditions which have this presentation and have a high priority. A number of general discriminators are used including *Life Threat*, *Pain* and *Temperature*. Specific discriminators have been included to indicate high chance of more serious pathology. If the patient is under 28 days, the Unwell newborn chart should be used

Specific discriminators	Explanation
Stridor	This may be an inspiratory or expiratory noise or both. Stridor is heard best on breathing with the mouth open
Drooling	Saliva running from the mouth as a result of being unable to swallow
Known or likely immunosuppression	Any patient who is known or likely to be immunosuppressed including those on immunosuppressive drugs (including long-term steroids)
Special risk of infection	Known exposure to a dangerous pathogen or travel to an area with an identified, current serious infectious risk
Possible sepsis	Suspected sepsis in patients who present with altered mental state, low blood pressure (Systolic less than 100) or raised respiratory rate (rate more than 22). In children, age specific physiological tools should be used to determine if possibly septic
Rapid onset	Onset within the preceding 12 hours
History of recent foreign travel	Recent significant foreign travel (within 2 weeks)

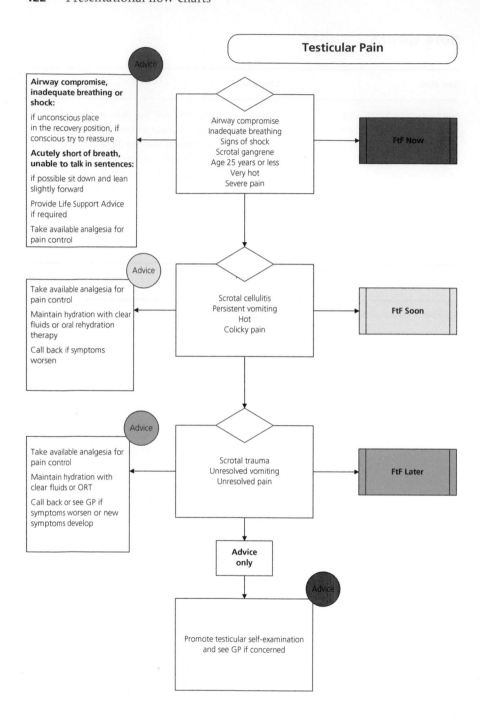

Testicular Pain

Airway compromise, inadequate breathing or shock:

if unconscious place in the recovery position, if conscious try to reassure

Acutely short of breath, unable to talk in sentences:

if possible sit down and lean slightly forward

Provide Life Support Advice if required

Take available analgesia for pain control

Airway compromise
Inadequate breathing
Signs of shock
Scrotal gangrene
Age 25 years or less
Very hot
Severe pain

FtF Now

Take available analgesia for pain control

Maintain hydration with clear fluids or oral rehydration therapy

Call back if symptoms worsen

Scrotal cellulitis
Persistent vomiting
Hot
Colicky pain

FtF Soon

Take available analgesia for pain control

Maintain hydration with clear fluids or ORT

Call back or see GP if symptoms worsen or new symptoms develop

Scrotal trauma
Unresolved vomiting
Unresolved pain

FtF Later

Advice only

Promote testicular self-examination and see GP if concerned

Advice

Testicular pain

See also	Chart notes
Abdominal pain Unwell newborn	This is a presentation-defined flow diagram. Testicular pain may have a number of pathologies, the most urgent of which is testicular torsion. A number of general discriminators are used including *Life Threat*, *Pain* and *Temperature*. Specific discriminators included in the 'face to face Now' and 'face to face Soon' category are designed to indicate those patients who have a high chance or torsion of the testes and the most severe infections. If the patient is under 28 days, the Unwell newborn chart should be used

Specific discriminators	Explanation
Scrotal gangrene	Dead blackened skin around the scrotum and groin. Early gangrene may not be black but may appear like a full thickness burn with or without flaking
Age 25 years or less	A person aged less than 25 years
Scrotal cellulitis	Redness and swelling around the scrotum
Persistent vomiting	Vomiting that is continuous or that occurs without any respite between episodes
Colicky pain	Pain that comes and goes in waves. Renal colic tends to come and go over 20 minutes or so
Scrotal trauma	Any recent physically traumatic event involving the scrotum

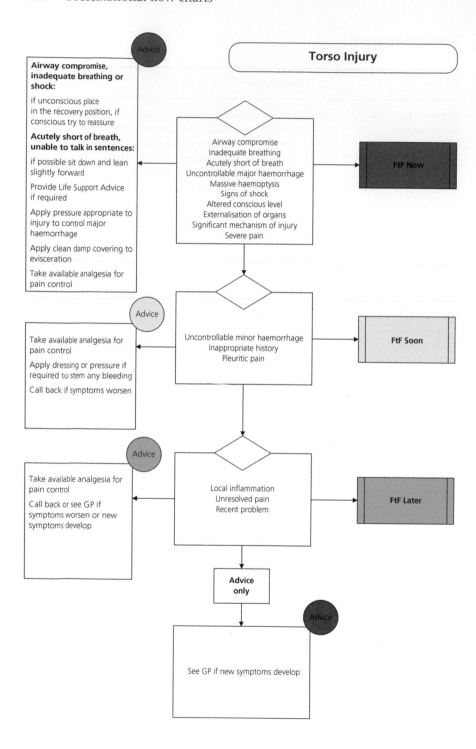

Torso Injury

Advice

Airway compromise, inadequate breathing or shock:

if unconscious place in the recovery position, if conscious try to reassure

Acutely short of breath, unable to talk in sentences:

if possible sit down and lean slightly forward

Provide Life Support Advice if required

Apply pressure appropriate to injury to control major haemorrhage

Apply clean damp covering to evisceration

Take available analgesia for pain control

Airway compromise
Inadequate breathing
Acutely short of breath
Uncontrollable major haemorrhage
Massive haemoptysis
Signs of shock
Altered conscious level
Externalisation of organs
Significant mechanism of injury
Severe pain

FtF Now

Advice

Take available analgesia for pain control

Apply dressing or pressure if required to stem any bleeding

Call back if symptoms worsen

Uncontrollable minor haemorrhage
Inappropriate history
Pleuritic pain

FtF Soon

Advice

Take available analgesia for pain control

Call back or see GP if symptoms worsen or new symptoms develop

Local inflammation
Unresolved pain
Recent problem

FtF Later

Advice only

Advice

See GP if new symptoms develop

Torso injury

See also	Chart notes
Assault Major trauma Wounds	This is a presentation-defined flow diagram designed to allow accurate prioritisation of patients who have suffered injuries to the front or back of the chest and abdomen. A number of general discriminators are used including *Life Threat*, *Haemorrhage* and *Pain*. Specific discriminators have been used to allow identification of patients who suffer from less obvious but severe internal injury. These would include patients who are acutely short of breath and those with a history suggestive of significant trauma

Specific discriminators	Explanation
Massive haemoptysis	Coughing up large amounts of fresh or clotted blood. Not to be confused with streaks of blood in saliva
Acutely short of breath	Shortness of breath that comes on suddenly or a sudden exacerbation of chronic shortness of breath
Externalisation of organs	Herniation or frank extrusion of internal organs
Significant mechanism of injury	Penetrating injuries (stab or gunshot) and injuries with high energy transfer
Inappropriate history	When the history (story) given does not explain the physical findings, it is termed inappropriate. This is important as it is a marker of safeguarding concerns in both adults and children
Pleuritic pain	A sharp, localised pain in the chest that worsens on breathing, coughing or sneezing
Local inflammation	Local inflammation will involve pain, swelling and redness confined to a particular site or area

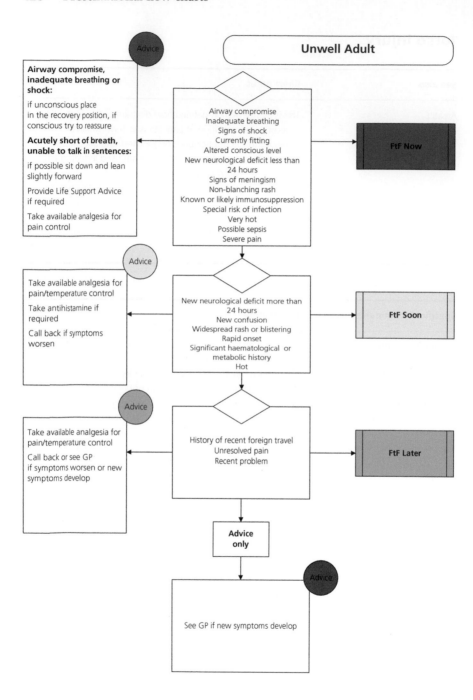

Advice

Unwell Adult

Airway compromise, inadequate breathing or shock:

if unconscious place in the recovery position, if conscious try to reassure

Acutely short of breath, unable to talk in sentences:

if possible sit down and lean slightly forward

Provide Life Support Advice if required

Take available analgesia for pain control

Airway compromise
Inadequate breathing
Signs of shock
Currently fitting
Altered conscious level
New neurological deficit less than 24 hours
Signs of meningism
Non-blanching rash
Known or likely immunosuppression
Special risk of infection
Very hot
Possible sepsis
Severe pain

FtF Now

Advice

Take available analgesia for pain/temperature control

Take antihistamine if required

Call back if symptoms worsen

New neurological deficit more than 24 hours
New confusion
Widespread rash or blistering
Rapid onset
Significant haematological or metabolic history
Hot

FtF Soon

Advice

Take available analgesia for pain/temperature control

Call back or see GP if symptoms worsen or new symptoms develop

History of recent foreign travel
Unresolved pain
Recent problem

FtF Later

Advice only

Advice

See GP if new symptoms develop

Unwell adult

See also	Chart notes
Collapsed adult	This is a non-specific presentation-defined flow diagram. A number of general discriminators are used including *Life Threat*, *Conscious Level*, *Pain* and *Temperature*. Specific discriminators have been included to ensure that patients with, for example, meningococcaemia are placed in appropriate category

Specific discriminators	Explanation
New neurological deficit less than 24 hours	Any loss of neurological function that has come on within the previous 24 hours. This might include altered or lost sensation, weakness of the limbs (either transiently or permanently) and alterations in bladder or bowel function
Signs of meningism	Classically a stiff neck together with headache and photophobia
Non-blanching rash	A rash that does not blanch (go white) when pressure is applied to it. Often tested using a glass tumbler to apply pressure as any colour change can be observed through the bottom of the tumbler
Known or likely immunosuppression	Any patient who is known to be immunosuppressed including those on immunosuppressive drugs (including long-term steroids)
Special risk of infection	Known exposure to a dangerous pathogen or travel to an area with an identified, current serious infectious risk
Possible sepsis	Suspected sepsis in patients who present with altered mental state, low blood pressure (Systolic less than 100) or raised respiratory rate (rate more than 22). In children, age specific physiological tools should be used to determine if possibly septic
New neurological deficit more than 24 hours	Any loss of neurological function including altered or lost sensation, weakness of the limbs (either transiently or permanently) and alterations in bladder or bowel function
New confusion	Patients with new onset confusion
Widespread rash or blistering	Any rash or blistering eruption covering more than 10% of the body surface area
Rapid onset	Onset within the preceding 12 hours
Significant haematological or metabolic history	A patient with a significant haematological condition; or a congenital metabolic disorder that is known to deteriorate rapidly
History of recent foreign travel	Recent significant foreign travel (within 2 weeks)

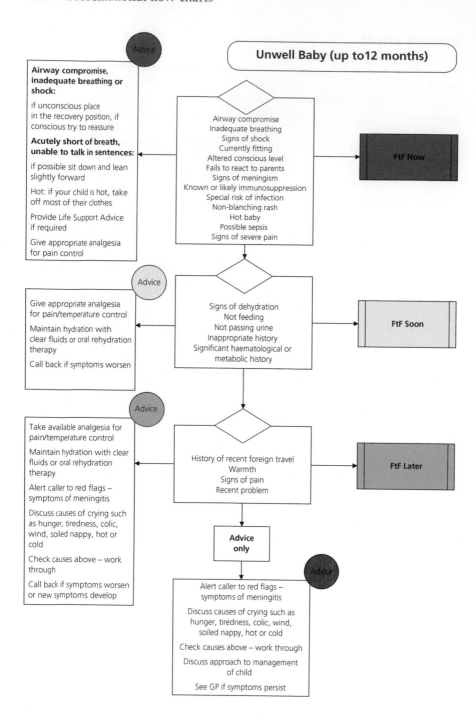

Unwell Baby (up to 12 months)

Airway compromise
Inadequate breathing
Signs of shock
Currently fitting
Altered conscious level
Fails to react to parents
Signs of meningism
Known or likely immunosuppression
Special risk of infection
Non-blanching rash
Hot baby
Possible sepsis
Signs of severe pain

FtF Now

Advice

Airway compromise, inadequate breathing or shock:

if unconscious place in the recovery position, if conscious try to reassure

Acutely short of breath, unable to talk in sentences:

if possible sit down and lean slightly forward

Hot: if your child is hot, take off most of their clothes

Provide Life Support Advice if required

Give appropriate analgesia for pain control

Advice

Signs of dehydration
Not feeding
Not passing urine
Inappropriate history
Significant haematological or metabolic history

FtF Soon

Give appropriate analgesia for pain/temperature control

Maintain hydration with clear fluids or oral rehydration therapy

Call back if symptoms worsen

Advice

History of recent foreign travel
Warmth
Signs of pain
Recent problem

FtF Later

Take available analgesia for pain/temperature control

Maintain hydration with clear fluids or oral rehydration therapy

Alert caller to red flags – symptoms of meningitis

Discuss causes of crying such as hunger, tiredness, colic, wind, soiled nappy, hot or cold

Check causes above – work through

Call back if symptoms worsen or new symptoms develop

Advice only

Advice

Alert caller to red flags – symptoms of meningitis

Discuss causes of crying such as hunger, tiredness, colic, wind, soiled nappy, hot or cold

Check causes above – work through

Discuss approach to management of child

See GP if symptoms persist

Unwell baby (up to 12 months)

	Chart notes
Unwell newborn	This is a presentation-defined flow diagram designed to allow accurate prioritisation of babies who present with non-specific illness. A number of general discriminators are used including *Life Threat*, *Conscious Level*, *Pain* and *Temperature*. A number of specific discriminators have been included to allow identification of more serious pathology such as meningococcaemia. **If the patient is under 28 days, the unwell newborn chart should be used**

Specific discriminators	Explanation
Fails to react to parents	Failure to react in any way to a parent's face or voice. Abnormal reactions and apparent lack of recognition of a parent are also worrying signs
Signs of meningism	Classically a stiff neck together with headache and photophobia
Known or likely immunosuppression	Any patient who is known or likely to be immunosuppressed including those on immunosuppressive drugs (including long-term steroids)
Special risk of infection	Known exposure to a dangerous pathogen, or travel to an area with an identified, current serious infectious risk
Possible sepsis	Suspected sepsis in patients who present with altered mental state, low blood pressure (Systolic less than 100) or raised respiratory rate (rate more than 22). In children, age specific physiological tools should be used to determine if possibly septic
Non-blanching rash	A rash that does not blanch (go white) when pressure is applied to it. Often tested using a glass tumbler to apply pressure as any colour change can be observed through the bottom of the tumbler
Signs of dehydration	These include dry tongue, sunken eyes, reduced skin turgor and, in small babies, a sunken anterior fontanelle. Usually associated with a low urine output
Not feeding	Children who do not take any solid or liquid (as appropriate) by mouth. Children who take the food but always vomit afterwards may also fulfil this criterion
Not passing urine	Failure to produce and pass urine. This may be difficult to judge in children (and the elderly) and reference to the number of nappies or pads used may be useful
Inappropriate history	When the history (story) given does not explain the physical findings, it is termed inappropriate. This is important as it is a marker of safeguarding concerns in both adults and children
Significant haematological or metabolic history	A patient with a significant haematological condition; or a congenital metabolic disorder that is known to deteriorate rapidly
History of recent foreign travel	Recent significant foreign travel (within 2 weeks)

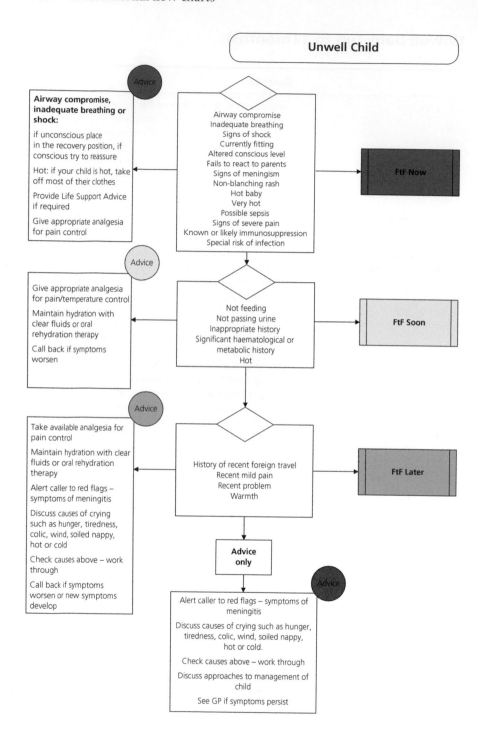

Unwell Child

Airway compromise, inadequate breathing or shock:

if unconscious place in the recovery position, if conscious try to reassure

Hot: if your child is hot, take off most of their clothes

Provide Life Support Advice if required

Give appropriate analgesia for pain control

Advice

Airway compromise
Inadequate breathing
Signs of shock
Currently fitting
Altered conscious level
Fails to react to parents
Signs of meningism
Non-blanching rash
Hot baby
Very hot
Possible sepsis
Signs of severe pain
Known or likely immunosuppression
Special risk of infection

FtF Now

Advice

Give appropriate analgesia for pain/temperature control

Maintain hydration with clear fluids or oral rehydration therapy

Call back if symptoms worsen

Not feeding
Not passing urine
Inappropriate history
Significant haematological or metabolic history
Hot

FtF Soon

Advice

Take available analgesia for pain control

Maintain hydration with clear fluids or oral rehydration therapy

Alert caller to red flags – symptoms of meningitis

Discuss causes of crying such as hunger, tiredness, colic, wind, soiled nappy, hot or cold

Check causes above – work through

Call back if symptoms worsen or new symptoms develop

History of recent foreign travel
Recent mild pain
Recent problem
Warmth

FtF Later

Advice only

Advice

Alert caller to red flags – symptoms of meningitis

Discuss causes of crying such as hunger, tiredness, colic, wind, soiled nappy, hot or cold.

Check causes above – work through

Discuss approaches to management of child

See GP if symptoms persist

Unwell child

See also	Chart notes
Crying baby Irritable child Worried parent	This is a presentation-defined flow diagram designed to allow accurate prioritisation of children **aged over 12 months** who present with non-specific illness. A number of general discriminators are used including *Life Threat*, *Conscious Level*, *Pain* and *Temperature*. A number of specific discriminators have been included to allow identification of more serious pathology such as meningococcaemia. If the patient is under 28 days, the Unwell newborn chart should be used

Specific discriminators	Explanation
Fails to react to parents	Failure to react in any way to a parent's face or voice. Abnormal reactions and apparent lack of recognition of a parent are also worrying signs
Special risk of infection	Known exposure to a dangerous pathogen, or travel to an area with an identified, current serious infectious risk
Signs of meningism	Classically a stiff neck together with headache and photophobia
Non-blanching rash	A rash that does not blanch (go white) when pressure is applied to it. Often tested using a glass tumbler to apply pressure as any colour change can be observed through the bottom of the tumbler
Possible sepsis	Suspected sepsis in patients who present with altered mental state, low blood pressure (Systolic less than 100) or raised respiratory rate (rate more than 22). In children, age specific physiological tools should be used to determine if possibly septic
Known or likely immunosuppression	Any patient who is known or likely to be immunosuppressed including those on immunosuppressive drugs (including long-term steroids)
Not feeding	Children who do not take any solid or liquid (as appropriate) by mouth. Children who take the food but always vomit afterwards may also fulfil this criterion
Not passing urine	Failure to produce and pass urine. This may be difficult to judge in children (and the elderly) and reference to the number of nappies or pads used may be useful
Inappropriate history	When the history (story) given does not explain the physical findings, it is termed inappropriate. This is important as it is a marker of safeguarding concerns in both adults and children
Significant haematological or metabolic history	A patient with a significant haematological condition; or a congenital metabolic disorder that is known to deteriorate rapidly
History of recent foreign travel	Recent significant foreign travel (within 2 weeks)

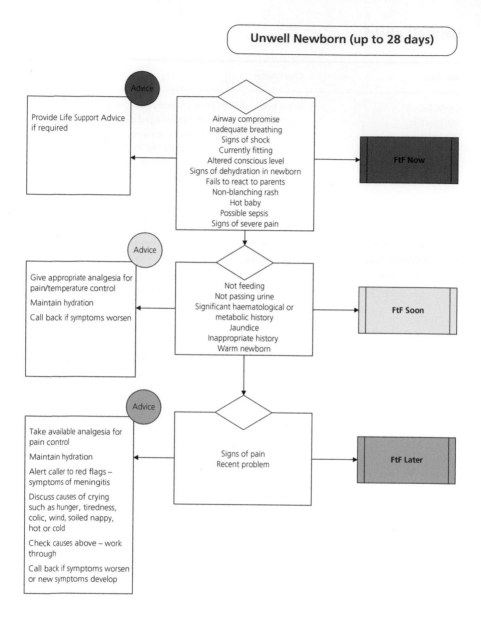

Unwell Newborn (up to 28 days)

Advice

Provide Life Support Advice if required

Airway compromise
Inadequate breathing
Signs of shock
Currently fitting
Altered conscious level
Signs of dehydration in newborn
Fails to react to parents
Non-blanching rash
Hot baby
Possible sepsis
Signs of severe pain

FtF Now

Advice

Give appropriate analgesia for pain/temperature control

Maintain hydration

Call back if symptoms worsen

Not feeding
Not passing urine
Significant haematological or metabolic history
Jaundice
Inappropriate history
Warm newborn

FtF Soon

Advice

Take available analgesia for pain control

Maintain hydration

Alert caller to red flags – symptoms of meningitis

Discuss causes of crying such as hunger, tiredness, colic, wind, soiled nappy, hot or cold

Check causes above – work through

Call back if symptoms worsen or new symptoms develop

Signs of pain
Recent problem

FtF Later

Unwell newborn (up to 28 days)

Chart notes

This is a presentation-defined flow diagram designed to allow accurate prioritisation of **newborns (up to 28 days)** who present with non-specific illness. A number of general discriminators are used including *Life Threat*, *Conscious Level*, *Pain* and *Temperature*. A number of specific discriminators have been included to allow identification of more serious pathology such as meningococcaemia.

Specific discriminators	Explanation
Signs of dehydration	These include dry tongue, sunken eyes, reduced skin turgor and, in small babies, a sunken anterior fontanelle. Usually associated with a low urine output
Fails to react to parents	Failure to react in any way to a parent's face or voice. Abnormal reactions and apparent lack of recognition of a parent are also worrying signs
Special risk of infection	Known exposure to a dangerous pathogen, or travel to an area with an identified, current serious infectious risk
Non-blanching rash	A rash that does not blanch (go white) when pressure is applied to it. Often tested using a glass tumbler to apply pressure as any colour change can be observed through the bottom of the tumbler
Signs of severe pain	Young children and babies in severe pain cannot complain. They will usually cry out continuously and inconsolably and be tachycardic. They may well exhibit signs such as pallor and sweating
Possible sepsis	Suspected sepsis in patients who present with altered mental state, low blood pressure (Systolic less than 100) or raised respiratory rate (rate more than 22). In children, age specific physiological tools should be used to determine if possibly septic
Not feeding	Children who do not take any solid or liquid (as appropriate) by mouth. Children who take the food but always vomit afterwards may also fulfil this criterion
Not passing urine	Failure to produce and pass urine. This may be difficult to judge in children (and the elderly) and reference to the number of nappies or pads used may be useful
Significant haematological or metabolic history	A patient with a significant haematological condition; or a congenital metabolic disorder that is known to deteriorate rapidly
Jaundice	Neonatal jaundice
Inappropriate history	When the history (story) given does not explain the physical findings, it is termed inappropriate. This is important as it is a marker of safeguarding concerns in both adults and children
History of recent foreign travel	Recent significant foreign travel (within 2 weeks)

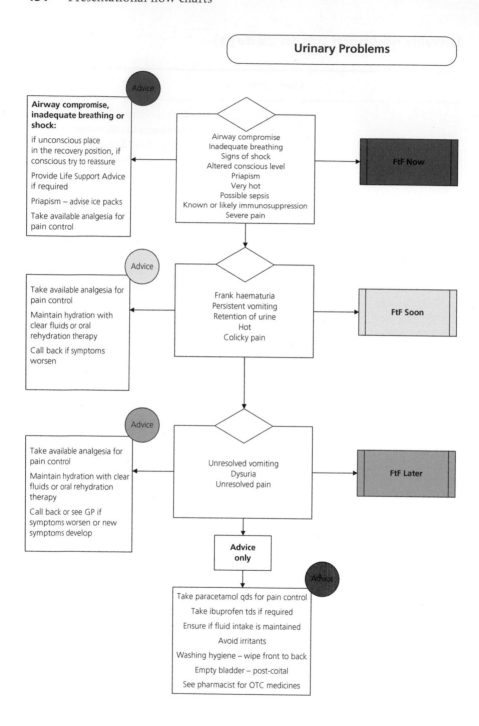

Urinary Problems

Advice

Airway compromise, inadequate breathing or shock:

if unconscious place in the recovery position, if conscious try to reassure

Provide Life Support Advice if required

Priapism – advise ice packs

Take available analgesia for pain control

Airway compromise
Inadequate breathing
Signs of shock
Altered conscious level
Priapism
Very hot
Possible sepsis
Known or likely immunosuppression
Severe pain

FtF Now

Advice

Take available analgesia for pain control

Maintain hydration with clear fluids or oral rehydration therapy

Call back if symptoms worsen

Frank haematuria
Persistent vomiting
Retention of urine
Hot
Colicky pain

FtF Soon

Advice

Take available analgesia for pain control

Maintain hydration with clear fluids or oral rehydration therapy

Call back or see GP if symptoms worsen or new symptoms develop

Unresolved vomiting
Dysuria
Unresolved pain

FtF Later

Advice only

Advice

Take paracetamol qds for pain control
Take ibuprofen tds if required
Ensure if fluid intake is maintained
Avoid irritants
Washing hygiene – wipe front to back
Empty bladder – post-coital
See pharmacist for OTC medicines

Urinary problems

See also	Chart notes
Sexually acquired infection Testicular pain	This is a presentation-defined flow diagram. A lot of patients who present with urinary problems complain of pain and some may have serious underlying pathology. A number of general discriminators are used including *Life Threat*, *Pain* and *Temperature*. Specific discriminators have been included to ensure that patients suffering from urinary retention and those with infections are included in appropriate categories. If the patient is under 28 days, the Unwell newborn chart should be used

Specific discriminators	Explanation
Priapism	Sustained penile erection
Possible sepsis	Suspected sepsis in patients who present with altered mental state, low blood pressure (Systolic less than 100) or raised respiratory rate (rate more than 22). In children, age specific physiological tools should be used to determine if possibly septic
Known or likely immunosuppression	Any patient who is known to be immunosuppressed including those on immunosuppressive drugs (including long-term steroids)
Frank haematuria	Red discolouration of the urine caused by blood
Persistent vomiting	Vomiting that is continuous or that occurs without any respite between episodes
Retention of urine	Inability to pass urine per urethra associated with an enlarged bladder. This condition is usually very painful unless there is altered sensation
Colicky pain	Pain that comes and goes in waves. Renal colic tends to come and go over 20 minutes or so
Dysuria	Pain or difficulty in passing urine. Pain is typically described as stinging or hot

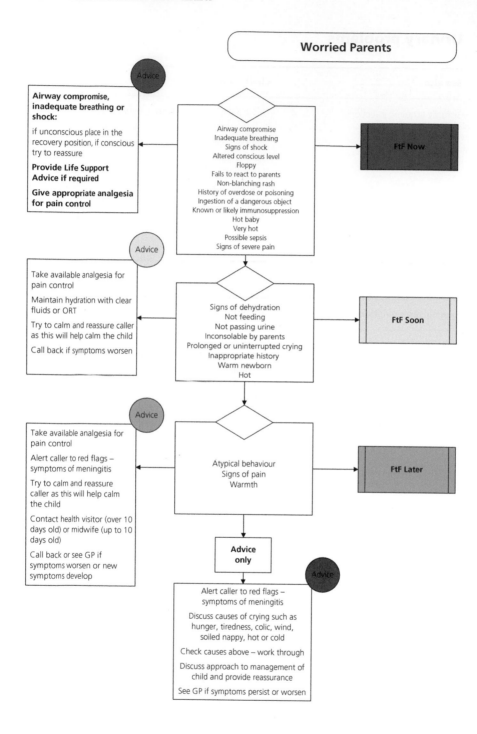

Worried Parents

Advice

Airway compromise, inadequate breathing or shock:

if unconscious place in the recovery position, if conscious try to reassure

Provide Life Support Advice if required

Give appropriate analgesia for pain control

Airway compromise
Inadequate breathing
Signs of shock
Altered conscious level
Floppy
Fails to react to parents
Non-blanching rash
History of overdose or poisoning
Ingestion of a dangerous object
Known or likely immunosuppression
Hot baby
Very hot
Possible sepsis
Signs of severe pain

FtF Now

Advice

Take available analgesia for pain control

Maintain hydration with clear fluids or ORT

Try to calm and reassure caller as this will help calm the child

Call back if symptoms worsen

Signs of dehydration
Not feeding
Not passing urine
Inconsolable by parents
Prolonged or uninterrupted crying
Inappropriate history
Warm newborn
Hot

FtF Soon

Advice

Take available analgesia for pain control

Alert caller to red flags – symptoms of meningitis

Try to calm and reassure caller as this will help calm the child

Contact health visitor (over 10 days old) or midwife (up to 10 days old)

Call back or see GP if symptoms worsen or new symptoms develop

Atypical behaviour
Signs of pain
Warmth

FtF Later

Advice only

Advice

Alert caller to red flags – symptoms of meningitis

Discuss causes of crying such as hunger, tiredness, colic, wind, soiled nappy, hot or cold

Check causes above – work through

Discuss approach to management of child and provide reassurance

See GP if symptoms persist or worsen

Worried parent

See also	Chart notes
Crying baby Irritable child Unwell child Unwell newborn	This is a presentation-defined flow diagram which has been designed to allow accurate prioritisation of children who are brought to the attention of the service because of parental worry. Parents know their children better than anyone else, and although many of these children will not have serious pathology, it is essential that these presentations are taken seriously A number of general discriminators are used including *Life Threat*, *Conscious Level*, *Pain* and *Temperature*. Specific discriminators have been added to the chart to allow identification of more serious pathologies which are apparent or may potentially exist If the patient is under 28 days, the unwell newborn chart should be used.

Specific discriminators	Explanation
Floppy	Parents may describe their children as floppy. Tone is generally reduced – the most noticeable sign is often lolling of the head
Fails to react to parents	Failure to react in any way to a parent's face or voice. Abnormal reactions and apparent lack of recognition of a parent are also worrying signs
Non-blanching rash	A rash that does not blanch (go white) when pressure is applied to it. Often tested using a glass tumbler to apply pressure as any colour change can be observed through the bottom of the tumbler
History of overdose or poisoning	This information may come from others or may be deduced if medication is missing
Known or likely immunosuppression	Any patient who is known to be immunosuppressed including those on immunosuppressive drugs (including long-term steroids)
Ingestion of a dangerous object	Ingestion of a dangerous or potentially dangerous foreign object e.g. button battery, magnets or razor blades which may be a potential threat to life
Possible sepsis	Suspected sepsis in patients who present with altered mental state, low blood pressure (Systolic less than 100) or raised respiratory rate (rate more than 22). In children, age specific physiological tools should be used to determine if possibly septic
Signs of dehydration	These include dry tongue, sunken eyes, decreased skin turgor and, in small babies, a sunken anterior fontanelle. Usually associated with a low urine output
Not feeding	Children who do take any solid or liquid (as appropriate) by mouth. Children who take the food but always vomit afterwards may also fulfil this criterion
Not passing urine	Failure to produce and pass urine. This may be difficult to judge in children (and the elderly) and reference to the number of nappies or pads used may be useful
Inconsolable by parents	Children whose crying or distress does not respond to attempts by their parents to comfort them fulfil this criterion
Prolonged or uninterrupted crying	A child who has cried continuously for 2 hours or more fulfils this criterion
Inappropriate history	When the history (story) given does not explain the physical findings, it is termed inappropriate. This is important as it is a marker of safeguarding concerns in both adults and children
Atypical behaviour	Children who behave in a way that is not usual in the given situation. The carers will often volunteer this information. Such children are often referred to as fractious or 'out of sorts'

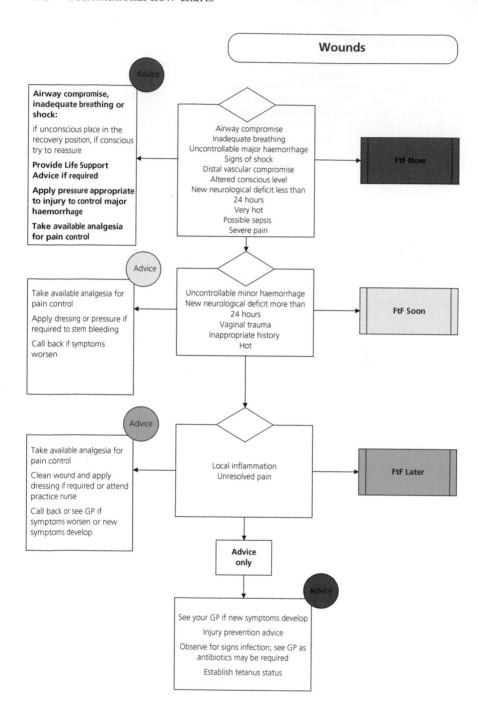

Wounds

Advice

Airway compromise, inadequate breathing or shock:

if unconscious place in the recovery position, if conscious try to reassure

Provide Life Support Advice if required

Apply pressure appropriate to injury to control major haemorrhage

Take available analgesia for pain control

Airway compromise
Inadequate breathing
Uncontrollable major haemorrhage
Signs of shock
Distal vascular compromise
Altered conscious level
New neurological deficit less than 24 hours
Very hot
Possible sepsis
Severe pain

FtF Now

Advice

Take available analgesia for pain control

Apply dressing or pressure if required to stem bleeding

Call back if symptoms worsen

Uncontrollable minor haemorrhage
New neurological deficit more than 24 hours
Vaginal trauma
Inappropriate history
Hot

FtF Soon

Advice

Take available analgesia for pain control

Clean wound and apply dressing if required or attend practice nurse

Call back or see GP if symptoms worsen or new symptoms develop

Local inflammation
Unresolved pain

FtF Later

Advice only

Advice

See your GP if new symptoms develop

Injury prevention advice

Observe for signs infection; see GP as antibiotics may be required

Establish tetanus status

Wounds

See also	Chart notes
Assault	This is a presentation-defined flow diagram. Many patients present to emergency care suffering from wounds of various nature. These vary from severe life-threatening lacerations to minor abrasions. This chart is designed to allow an accurate prioritisation of these patients.
	A number of general discriminators have been used including *Life Threat*, *Haemorrhage* and *Pain*. Specific discriminators have been included to allow identification of patients with signs and symptoms suggesting injuries which pose a threat to function

Specific discriminators	Explanation
Distal vascular compromise	There will be a combination of pallor, coldness, altered sensation and pain with or without absent pulses distal to the injury
New neurological deficit less than 24 hours	Any loss of neurological function that has come on within the previous 24 hours. This might include altered or lost sensation, weakness of the limbs (either transiently or permanently) and alterations in bladder or bowel function
Possible sepsis	Suspected sepsis in patients who present with altered mental state, low blood pressure (Systolic less than 100) or raised respiratory rate (rate more than 22). In children, age specific physiological tools should be used to determine if possibly septic
New neurological deficit more than 24 hours	Any loss of neurological function that has come on within the previous 24 hours. This might include altered or lost sensation, weakness of the limbs (either transiently or permanently) and alterations in bladder or bowel function
Vaginal trauma	Any history or other evidence of direct trauma to the vagina fulfils this criterion
Inappropriate history	When the history (story) given does not explain the physical findings, it is termed inappropriate. This is important as it is a marker of safeguarding concerns in both adults and children
Local inflammation	Local inflammation will involve pain, swelling and redness confined to a particular site or area

Discriminator and question dictionary

Discriminator	Questions	Definition
Abdominal pain	Do you have pain in your tummy?	Any pain felt in the abdomen. Abdominal pain associated with back pain may indicate abdominal aortic aneurysm, whilst association with PV bleeding may indicate ectopic pregnancy or miscarriage
Abrupt onset	How long ago did it start? When did it come on? Did it come on suddenly?	Onset within seconds or minutes. May cause waking from sleep
Acute chemical eye injury		Any substance splashed into or placed into the eye within the past 12 hours that caused stinging, burning or reduced vision should be assumed to have caused chemical injury
Acute complete loss of vision		Loss of vision in one or both eyes within the preceding 24 hours which has not returned to normal
Acute onset after injury	Did this start after you *fell/ were hit*, etc.? When did this start?	Onset of symptoms immediately within 24 hours of a physically traumatic event

Emergency Triage: Telephone triage and advice, First Edition. Updated version 1.7, 2023.
Edited by Janet Marsden, Mark Newton, Jill Windle and Kevin Mackway-Jones.
© 2016 John Wiley & Sons, Ltd. Published 2016 by John Wiley & Sons, Ltd.

Discriminator	Questions	Definition
Acutely avulsed tooth	When did your tooth come out? Was this the result of injury? Is it complete with a root?	A tooth that has been avulsed intact within the previous 24 hours
Acutely short of breath	Have you suddenly become short of breath? Are you more short of breath than normal?	Shortness of breath that comes on suddenly or a sudden exacerbation of chronic shortness of breath
Age 25 years or less	How old are you?	A person aged less than 25 years
Airway compromise	Are they awake? Are they struggling to breathe? Can they get their breath in? Do they make a gurgling sound when they breathe?	An airway may be compromised either because it cannot be kept open or because the airway protective reflexes (that stop inhalation) have been lost. Failure to keep the airway open will result either in intermittent total obstruction or in partial obstruction. This will manifest itself as snoring or bubbling sounds during breathing
Altered conscious level	Do they open their eyes or move when you speak to them or gently shake their shoulders? Have they had alcohol? Have they had alcohol?	Not fully alert. Either responding to voice or pain only or unresponsive
Altered facial sensation		Any alteration of sensation on the face
Aortic pain		The onset of symptoms is sudden and the leading symptom is severe abdominal or chest pain. The pain may be described as sharp, stabbing or ripping in character. Classically aortic chest pain is felt around the sternum and then radiates to the shoulder blades, aortic abdominal pain is felt in the centre of the abdomen and radiates to the back. The pain may get better or even vanish and then recur elsewhere. Over time, pain may also be felt in the arms, neck, lower jaw, stomach or hips

(Continued)

(*Continued*)

Discriminator	Questions	Definition
Apparently hallucinating	Have you been hearing or seeing things that no one else has seen or heard? Is this the first time you have heard voices? What have the voices been telling you to do?	Patients who are apparently hallucinating may appear distracted and may appear to react to stimuli (primarily visual and auditory) that are not apparent to anyone else
Atypical behaviour	Is he behaving normally? Is he listless? Is he 'out of sorts'?	Children who are behaving in a way that is not usual in the given situation. The carers will often volunteer this information. Such children are often referred to as fractious or 'out of sorts'
Auricular haematoma	Have you had a blow on your ear? Did your ear swell up after you were hit on it? Is it painful?	A tense haematoma (usually post traumatic) in the outer ear
Black or redcurrant stool	What does the stool look like?	Any blackness fulfils the criteria of black stool while a dark red stool, classically seen in intussusceptions, is redcurrant stool
Bleeding disorder	Do you know of any reason why your blood doesn't clot normally?	Congenital or acquired bleeding disorder
Cardiac pain	Where is the pain? Have you had pain like this before? What is it like? Does it go to your arm or neck?	Classically, a severe dull 'gripping' or 'heavy' pain in the centre of the chest, radiating to the left arm or to the neck. May be associated with sweating and nausea
Chest injury	Have you injured your chest?	Any injury to the area below the clavicles and above the level of the lowest rib. Injury to the lower part of the chest can cause underlying damage to abdominal organs
Colicky pain	Do you have pain? Does it come and go in waves?	Pain that comes and goes in waves. Renal colic tends to come and go over 20 minutes or so
Current palpitation		A feeling of the heart racing (often described as a fluttering) that is still present
Currently fitting	Are they having a fit? What do they look like at the moment? Are their limbs jerking or shaking?	Patients who are in the tonic or clonic stages of a grand mal convulsion and patients currently experiencing partial fits
Deformity	Does it look the normal shape?	This will always be subjective. Abnormal angulation or rotation is implied
Diplopia		Double vision that resolves when one eye is closed

Discriminator	Questions	Definition
Direct trauma to the back	Have you been hit on your back? What exactly happened?	This may be top to bottom (loading), for instance, when someone falls and lands on their feet, bending (forwards, backwards or to the side) or twisting
Direct trauma to the neck	Have you been hit on your neck? What exactly happened?	This may be top to bottom (loading), for instance, when something falls on the head, bending (forwards, backwards or to the side) or twisting, or distracting such as in hanging
Discharge		In the context of sexually acquired infection, this is any discharge from the penis or abnormal discharge from the vagina
Discharged from mental health services within the past 15 days	Have you been recently discharged from any mental health services in the past 15 days?	Any patient who has been discharged from an active period of care under mental health services (in hospital or in the community) within the past 15 days
Distal vascular compromise	Does the limb look a different colour below the injury or when you compare it to the other side? Is the far part limb/area pale or blue? Is the far part of the limb/area pale?	There will be a combination of pallor, coldness, altered sensation and pain with or without absent pulses distal to the injury
Drooling	Is the spit dribbling from their mouth?	Saliva running from the mouth as a result of being unable to swallow
Dysuria	Does it burn or sting when you pass urine?	Pain or difficulty in passing urine. Pain is typically described as stinging or hot
Electrical injury	Have you had an electric shock?	Any injury caused or possibly caused by electric current. This includes AC and DC and both artificial and natural sources

(Continued)

(Continued)

Discriminator	Questions	Definition
Exhaustion		Exhausted patients appear to reduce the effort they make to breathe despite continuing respiratory insufficiency. This is pre-terminal
Externalisation of organs	Can you see their guts hanging out?	Herniation or frank extrusion of internal organs
Facial oedema	Is your face swollen? Is it swollen in a particular place or all over? How swollen is it?	Diffuse swelling around the face usually involving the lips
Fails to react to parents	Does he react to you at all? Is the reaction normal?	Failure to react in any way to a parents face or voice. Abnormal reactions and apparent lack of recognition of a parent are also worrying signs
Floppy	Are they floppy?	Parents may describe their children as floppy. Tone is generally reduced – the most noticeable sign is often lolling of the head
Foreign body sensation		A sensation of something in the eye, often expressed as scraping or grittiness
Frank haematuria	Is there blood in your urine? Is your urine red?	Red discolouration of the urine caused by blood
Gross deformity		This will always be subjective. Gross and abnormal angulation or rotation is implied
Headache	Do you have a headache?	Any pain around the head that is not related to a particular anatomical structure. Facial pain is not included
Head injury	Have you banged your head? Have you been hit on the head?	Any traumatic event involving the head
Heavy PV blood loss	How much blood are you losing? How many towels are you using? Is this normal for you?	PV loss is extremely difficult to assess. The presence of large clots or constant blood flow fulfils this criterion. The use of a large number of sanitary towels is suggestive of heavy loss

Discriminator	Questions	Definition
High blood pressure	Do you have high blood pressure? Are you taking medicine for high blood pressure?	A history of raised blood pressure or a raised blood pressure on examination
High lethality		Lethality is the potential of the substance taken to cause harm. Advice from a poisons centre may be required to establish the level of risk of serious illness or death. If in doubt, assume a high risk
High lethality envenomation		Lethality is the potential of the envenomation to cause harm. Local knowledge may allow identification of the venomous creature, but advice may be required. If in doubt assume a high risk
High lethality chemical		Lethality is the potential of the chemical to cause harm. Advice may be required to establish the level of risk. If in doubt, assume high risk
High risk of further self-harm	Are you actively harming yourself at the moment or planning to harm yourself in any way? Can I ask what you have used/are planning on using? Do you have access to that at the moment?	An initial view of the risk of harm to self can be formed by considering the patient's behaviour. Patients who are threatening to harm themselves and who are actively seeking the means to do so are at high risk
High risk of leaving before assessment	Are you able to wait for someone to arrive so they can assess you?	Active, credible threats to leave prior to assessment pose a high risk
High risk of self-harm	Are you actively harming yourself at the moment or planning to harm yourself in any way? Can I ask what you have used/are planning on using? Do you have access to that at the moment?	An initial view of the risk of harm to self can be formed by considering the patient's behaviour. Patients who are threatening to harm themselves and who are actively seeking the means to do so are at high risk

(Continued)

(Continued)

Discriminator	Questions	Definition
High risk to others	Speech patterns would be determined by talking to the patient however in order to assess behaviour and posture it may be necessary to ask questions to someone who is with the patient if possible. Have you been physically harmed? Do you feel the patient is a risk to you?	An initial view of the risk of harm to others can be judged by assessing posture (tense, clenched), speech (loud, using threatening words) loud background noise can be an indicator and motor behaviour (restless, pacing, lunging at others). High risk should be assumed if weapons and potential victims are available and no controls are already in place
History of acutely vomiting blood	Have you vomited any blood? Have you vomited up any brown stuff?	Frank haematemesis, vomiting of altered blood (coffee ground) or of blood mixed in the vomit within the past 24 hours
History of head injury	Have you banged your head? Have you been hit on the head?	A history of a recent physically traumatic event involving the head. Usually this will be reported by the patient but, if the patient has been unconscious, this history should be sought from a reliable witness
History of overdose or poisoning		This information may come from others or may be deduced if medication is missing
History of recent foreign travel	Have you travelled abroad lately? Where have you been?	Recent significant foreign travel (within 2 weeks)
History of trauma	Have you hurt yourself? Have you fallen or been involved in an accident?	A history of a recent physically traumatic event
History of unconsciousness	Were you (they) unconscious? Have you (they) been knocked out?	There may be a reliable witness who can state whether the patient was unconscious (and for how long). If not, a patient who is unable to remember the incident should be assumed to have been unconscious

Discriminator	Questions	Definition
Hot	Have you taken your temperature? What is it? Do you feel hot?	If the skin feels hot, the person is clinically said to be hot. A temperature of 38.5°C and greater is hot. Other clinical features of pyrexia should be taken into account.
Hot baby		If the skin is hot, the child is clinically said to be hot. The temperature should be taken as soon as possible – a temperature of 38.5°C and greater is hot. A baby is a child less than 1 year old
Hot joint	Is (are) your joint(s) hot to touch?	Any warmth around a joint fulfils this criterion. Often accompanied by redness
Hyperglycaemia		Glucose greater than 17 mmol/l
Hypoglycaemia		Glucose less than 3 mmol/l
In active labour	Are you getting contractions? Do you feel labour has started?	A woman who is having regular and frequent painful contractions
Inadequate breathing	Are they breathing? What is the colour of their lips and tongue?	Patients who are failing to breathe well enough to maintain adequate oxygenation have inadequate breathing. There may be an increased work of breathing, signs of inadequate breathing or exhaustion
Inappropriate history		When the history (story) given does not explain the physical findings, it is termed inappropriate. This is important as it is a marker of safeguarding concerns in both adults and children
Inconsolable by parents	Can you calm them down at all? Do they settle at all when you cuddle them?	Children whose crying or distress does not respond to attempts by their parents to comfort them

(Continued)

(Continued)

Discriminator	Questions	Definition
Ingestion of a dangerous object		Ingestion of a dangerous or potentially dangerous foreign object e.g. button battery, magnets or razor blades which may be a potential threat to life
Inhalational injury	Were they (you) confined in a place that was filled with smoke? Is there any soot in the nostrils or mouth?	A history of being confined in a smoke filled space is the most reliable indicator of smoke inhalation. Carbon deposits around the mouth and nose and hoarse voice may be present. History is also the most reliable way of diagnosing inhalation of chemicals – there will not necessarily be any signs
Jaundice		Neonatal jaundice
Known abdominal or aortic aneurysm	Have you (has the patient) ever had investigations for an aneurysm in your belly?	The patient is reported to have an abdominal or aortic aneurysm
Known or likely immunosuppression	Do you take any medicines? What are they? Do you have any illnesses that affect your immunity?	Any patient who is known or likely to be immunosuppressed including those on immunosuppressive drugs (including long term steroids)
Lack of medication causing exacerbation or relapse of condition		Lack of regular medications such as insulin which may cause exacerbation or relapse of condition if not obtained soon
Likely to require admission under mental health legislation	This will be subjective based on responses to the questions you have already asked	Patients with significant psychiatric symptoms who are likely to require admission under mental health legislation
Local inflammation	Is it red? Is it warm to touch?	Local inflammation will involve pain, swelling and redness confined to a particular site or area
Lower abdominal pain		Any pain felt in the abdomen; association with PV bleeding may indicate ectopic pregnancy or miscarriage
Marked distress	How do you feel? How are you?	Patients who are markedly physically or emotionally upset

Discriminator	Questions	Definition
Massive haemoptysis		Coughing up large amounts of fresh or clotted blood. Not to be confused with streaks of blood in saliva
Moderate aggression or agitation	This will be subjective based on the patients responses to other questions. If the caller has witnessed this in the patient before have they been able to verbally de-escalate Are you managing to de-escalate the situation/keep the patient calm?	Agitation or aggression that can usually be managed by verbal de-escalation without physical restraint
Moderate risk of further self harm	Are you actively harming yourself at the moment or planning to harm yourself in any way? Can I ask what you have used/ are planning on using? Do you have access to that at the moment?	An initial view of the risk of harm to self can be formed by considering the patient's behaviour. Patients without a significant history of self harm, who are not actively trying to harm themselves, but who profess the desire to harm themselves are at moderate risk
Moderate risk of harm to others	Speech patterns would be determined by talking to the patient however in order to assess behaviour and posture it may be necessary to ask questions to someone who is with the patient if possible.	An initial view of the risk of harm to others can be judged by assessing posture (tense, clenched), speech (loud, using threatening words) using threatening words) loud background noise can be an indicator and motor behaviour (restless, pacing, lunging at others). Moderate risk should be assumed if there is any indication of potential harm to others
Moderate risk of leaving before assessment	Are you able to wait for someone to arrive so they can assess you?	Threats to leave without any attempts to do so pose a moderate risk
Moderate risk of self harm	Are you actively harming yourself at the moment or planning to harm yourself in any way? Can I ask what you have used/ are planning on using? Do you have access to that at the moment?	An initial view of the risk of harm to self can be formed by considering the patient's behaviour. Patients without a significant history of self harm, who are not actively trying to harm themselves, but who profess the desire to harm themselves are at moderate risk
Moderate lethality chemical		Lethality is the potential of the chemical to cause harm. Advice may be required to establish the level of risk. If in doubt, assume a high risk.

(Continued)

(*Continued*)

Discriminator	Questions	Definition
Moderate lethality		Lethality is the potential of the substance taken to cause serious illness or death. Advice from a Poisons Centre may be required to establish the level of risk to the patient
Moderate lethality envenomation		Lethality is the potential of the envenomation to cause harm. Local knowledge may allow identification of the venomous creature, but advice may be required
New confusion	What has changed today? What is concerning you?	Patients with new onset confusion
New neurological deficit less than 24 hours old	Can you move all your arms and legs? Do you have any tingling or numbness? When did this start?	Any loss of neurological function that has come on within the previous 24 hours. This might include altered or lost sensation, weakness of the limbs (either transiently or permanently) and alterations in bladder or bowel function
New neurological deficit more than 24 hours old		Any loss of neurological function including altered or lost sensation, weakness of the limbs (either transiently or permanently) and alterations in bladder or bowel function
New onset of significant mental health symptoms	These symptoms you are experiencing today, are these completely new for you? Have you experienced them before?	Any new mental health symptoms not already taken into account
New symptoms of psychosis	Do you feel that people are out to get you or do you feel that you are going to be harmed Who do you think is going to harm you, is it a person or is it a thing Have you experienced these feelings before	Active new symptoms of psychosis with no insight such as hallucinations, delusions and/or paranoia
No improvement with own asthma medications	Have you got better since you took your treatment?	This history should be available from the patient. A failure to improve with bronchodilator therapy given by the GP or paramedic is equally significant

Discriminator	Questions	Definition
No medication available		No medication available
Non-blanching rash		A rash that does not blanch (go white) when pressure is applied to it. Often tested using a glass tumbler to apply pressure as any colour change can be observed through the bottom of the tumbler
Not distractible	Can you calm them down? Will they play with their toys? Will they take an interest in anything?	Children who are distressed by pain or other things who cannot be distracted by conversation or play
Not feeding	Are they managing to eat or drink? Can they take any fluids?	Children who will not take solid or liquid (as appropriate) by mouth. Children who will take the food but always vomit afterwards may also fulfil this criterion
Not passing urine	Are they passing any urine? Do they have any wet nappies? How many and is that normal for them?	Failure to produce and pass urine. This may be difficult to judge in children (and the elderly) and reference to the number of nappies or pads used may be useful
Oedema of the tongue	Is their tongue swollen?	Swelling of the tongue of any degree
Open fracture	Is there a cut near the broken bone? Is there bone sticking out?	All wounds in the vicinity of a fracture should be regarded with suspicion. If there is any possibility of communication between the wound and the fracture, then the fracture should be assumed to be open
Pain on joint movement	Does it hurt when you move your joint(s)?	This can be pain on both active (patient) movement or passive (examiner) movement
Passing fresh or altered blood PR	Are you passing blood from the back passage at the moment? What colour is it?	In active massive GI bleeding, dark red blood will be passed PR. As GI transit time increases, this becomes darker, eventually becoming melaena
Penetrating eye injury	Has it gone into your eye? Has anything stuck into your eye?	A recent physically traumatic event involving penetration of the globe

(Continued)

(*Continued*)

Discriminator	Questions	Definition
Persistent vomiting	Are you vomiting all the time? Does the vomiting ever stop?	Vomiting that is continuous or that occurs without any respite between episodes
Pleuritic pain	Is the pain sharp or dull? Is it worse on coughing? Is it worse on deep breathing?	A sharp pain in the chest worse on breathing, coughing or sneezing
Possible sepsis	Have you been recently unwell or had any recent infections? If yes, a sepsis screening tool should be applied.	Suspected sepsis in patients who present with altered mental state, low blood pressure (Systolic less than 100) or raised respiratory rate (rate more than 22). In children, age specific physiological tools should be used to determine if possibly septic.
Possibly pregnant	Could you be pregnant? When was your last period?	Any woman whose normal menstruation has failed to occur is possibly pregnant. Furthermore, any woman of childbearing age who has unprotected sex should be considered to be potentially pregnant
Presenting foetal parts	Can you see any part of the baby? Is the baby coming out?	Crowning or presentation of any other foetal part in the vagina
Priapism	Do you (they) have an erection?	Sustained penile erection
Productive cough		A cough which is productive of phlegm, whatever the colour
Prolonged or uninterrupted crying	How long have they been crying? Do they ever stop?	A child who has cried continuously for 2 hours or more
Purpura		A rash on any part of the body that is caused by small haemorrhages under the skin. A purpuric rash does not blanch (go white) when pressure is applied to it
PV blood loss	Is there any vaginal bleeding? Are you bleeding down below?	Any loss of blood PV
PV blood loss and 20 weeks pregnant or more		Any loss of blood PV in a woman known to be beyond the 20th week of pregnancy
Rapid onset	How quickly did it come on? Did it come on quickly? How quickly?	Onset within the preceding 12 hours

Discriminator	Questions	Definition
Recent hearing loss		Loss of hearing in one or both ears within the previous week
Recent problem	Has this come on in the last week? Has this got worse over the last week?	A problem arising in the last week
Recent reduced visual acuity		Any reduction in corrected visual acuity within the past 7 days
Recently given birth	Have you given birth within the last three months?	A woman who has given birth within the past 3 months
Red eye	Do you have redness of the eye? Is your eyeball red rather than white?	Any redness to the eye. A red eye may be painful or painless and may be complete or partial
Reduced foetal movements > 20 weeks	When did you last feel the baby move? How often does the baby usually move?	Absent or reduced foetal movements during the previous 12 hours in a woman known to be beyond the 20th week of pregnancy
Requesting post-coital contraception and unprotected sex 0–65 hours ago		Medication is required but there is a larger window of opportunity for obtaining it
Requesting post-coital contraception and unprotected sex 66–72 hours ago		There is a window of opportunity for post-coital contraception which best evidence suggests ends at 72 hours
Responds to pain		Response to a painful stimulus. Standard peripheral stimuli should be used – a pencil or pen is used to apply pressure to the finger nail bed.
Retention of urine	Can you pass water? When did you last pass water? Is it painful?	Inability to pass urine per urethra associated with an enlarged bladder. This condition is usually very painful unless there is altered sensation
Risk of continued contamination		If chemical exposure is likely to continue (usually due to lack of adequate decontamination) then this discriminator applies. Risks to health care workers must not be forgotten if this situation occurs

(*Continued*)

(Continued)

Discriminator	Questions	Definition
Safeguarding concerns	This will be subjective based on responses to the questions you have already asked	Any concerns for the welfare of the patient that arise from their vulnerability
Scrotal cellulitis	Is there any redness and warmth of the scrotum?	Redness and swelling around the scrotum
Scrotal gangrene	Is the scrotum black, discoloured or white and flaking?	Dead blackened skin around the scrotum and groin. Early gangrene may not be black but may appear like a full thickness burn with or without flaking
Scrotal trauma	Have you been kicked in the testicles?	Any recent physically traumatic event involving the scrotum
Self-harmed without other psychiatric disease	This will be subjective based on responses to the questions you have already asked	Patients who have harmed themselves (for the first or subsequent time) who do not have a mental health diagnosis
Severe aggression or agitation that may require restraint	Have you been physically harmed? Do you feel the patient is a risk to you? How will the patient react to the ambulance arriving? If you feel at risk remove yourself and others from the patient	Aggression and agitation of such a degree that restraint may be required at short notice to manage the risk of harm to self or others
Severe itch	Is the itch very bad? How bad is the itching?	An itch that is unbearable
Severe pain	Can they (you) describe how bad the pain is?	Pain that is unbearable – often described as the worst ever
Shoulder tip pain	Have you got any pain in your shoulder?	Pain felt in the tip of the shoulder. This often indicates diaphragmatic irritation
Significant cardiac history		A known recurrent dysrhythmia which has life-threatening effects is significant, as is a known cardiac condition that may deteriorate rapidly
Significant haematological or metabolic history		A patient with a significant haematological condition; or a congenital metabolic disorder that is known to deteriorate rapidly

Discriminator	Questions	Definition
Significant history of allergy	Have they ever had a severe reaction to anything? What happened?	A known sensitivity with severe reaction (e.g. to nuts or bee sting) is significant
Significant history of GI bleed		Any history of massive GI bleeding or of any GI bleed associated with oesophageal varices
Significant mechanism of injury	How did the injury occur?	Penetrating injuries (stab or gunshot) and injuries with high energy transfer
Significant psychiatric history	Do you have a psychiatrist? What for? Do you take any tranquillisers or other drugs?	A history of a major psychiatric illness or event
Significant respiratory history		A history of previous life threatening episodes of a respiratory condition (e.g. COPD) is significant as is brittle asthma
Signs of dehydration	Do you (they) have a dry tongue? Do you (they) look dry? Are you (they) passing as much urine as normal?	These include dry tongue, sunken eyes, decreased skin turgor and, in small babies, a sunken anterior fontanelle. Usually associated with a low urine output
Signs of meningism	Do you (they) have a stiff neck? Does the light hurt your (their) eyes?	Classically a stiff neck together with headache and photophobia
Signs of pain		Young children and babies in pain cannot complain. They will usually cry occasionally and may act atypically
Signs of severe pain	Do they look like they are in bad pain? Are they crying a lot? Are they screwing up their face? Are they drawing up their knees?	Young children and babies in severe pain cannot complain. They will usually cry out continuously and inconsolably and be tachycardic. They may well exhibit signs such as pallor and sweating
Signs of shock		Shock is inadequate delivery of oxygen to the tissues. The classic signs include sweating, pallor, tachycardia, hypotension and reduced conscious level

(Continued)

(*Continued*)

Discriminator	Questions	Definition
Smoke exposure	Were you (they) stuck in a smoke filled area?	Smoke inhalation should be assumed if the patient has been confined in a smoke-filled space. Physical signs such as oral or nasal soot are less reliable but significant if present
Special risk of infection		Known exposure to a dangerous pathogen or travel to an area with an identified, current serious infectious risk
Stridor	Do they make a noise in their throat when they breathe in or out? What does it sound like?	This may be an inspiratory or expiratory noise or both. Stridor is heard best on breathing with the mouth open
Swelling	Has it swollen up?	An abnormal increase in size
Temporal scalp tenderness		Tenderness on palpation over the temporal area (especially over the artery)
Testicular pain	Do you have pain in the testicles?	Pain in the testicles
Unable to feed	Are they feeding normally? Will they take any food?	This is usually reported by the parents. Children who will not take any solid or liquid (as appropriate) by mouth
Unable to talk in sentences	Are they so short of breath that they can't talk to you?	Patients who are so breathless that they cannot complete relatively short sentences in one breath
Unable to walk	Can they walk? Can they hobble about? Does it hurt to walk?	It is important to try and distinguish between patients who have pain and difficulty walking and those who *cannot* walk. Only the latter can be said to be unable to walk
Uncontrollable major haemorrhage	Are they bleeding a lot? Where is the blood coming from? Does the blood spurt out? Does the bleeding stop if you press on it?	A haemorrhage that is not rapidly controlled by the application of sustained direct pressure and which continues to bleed heavily or soak through large dressings quickly
Uncontrollable minor haemorrhage	Are they bleeding? Where is the blood coming from? Does the bleeding stop if you press on it?	A haemorrhage that is not rapidly controlled by the application of sustained direct pressure and which continues to bleed slightly or ooze

Discriminator	Questions	Definition
Unresolved itch		Itch that has not resolved despite waiting an appropriate time or taking appropriate medication
Unresolved pain		Pain which has not resolved despite waiting an appropriate time or being given appropriate analgesia
Unresolved rash		A rash that has not resolved despite waiting an appropriate time or being given appropriate therapy
Unresolved vomiting		Vomiting which has not resolved, despite any appropriate actions
Unresponsive child	Do they react to you at all? Can you waken them at all?	A child who fails to respond to either verbal or painful stimuli
Vaginal trauma		Any history or other evidence of direct trauma to the vagina
Vascular compromise	Does the limb look a different colour below the injury or when you compare it to the other side? Is the far part limb/area pale or blue? Is the far part of the limb/area pale?	There will be a combination of pallor, coldness, altered sensation and pain with or without absent pulses distal to the injury
Vertigo		An acute feeling of spinning or dizziness, possibly accompanied by nausea and vomiting
Very hot	Have they been shaking? Has the temperature been taken? What is it? How hot do they feel when you touch them? Do they say they are feeling cold?	If the skin feels very hot, the patient is clinically said to be very hot. This should be used with caution where a core temperature is not available and other signs of pyrexia should be taken into account. A temperature of 41°C or greater is very hot
Visible abdominal mass		A mass in the abdomen that is visible to the naked eye
Vomiting	Have you vomited since this happened?	Any emesis
Vomiting blood		Vomited blood may be fresh (bright or dark red) or coffee ground in appearance

(Continued)

(Continued)

Discriminator	Questions	Definition
Warm newborn		If the skin feels warm, the patient is clinically said to be warm. The temperature should be taken as soon as possible – a child of 28 days or under with a temperature of 37.5–38.4°C is warm
Warmth		If the skin feels warm, the patient is clinically said to be warm. The temperature should be taken as soon as possible – a temperature greater than 37.5°C is warm
Wheeze	Do they (you) sound wheezy when breathing?	This can be audible wheeze or a feeling of wheeze. Very severe airway obstruction is silent (no air can move)
Widespread discharge or blistering	Where are the blisters? How much of your body is covered by them? Are they discharging?	Any discharging or blistering eruption covering more than 10% body surface area
Widespread rash or blistering		Any rash or blistering eruption covering more than 10% of the body surface area
Withdrawal possible		Where the lack of medication will lead to symptoms of drug/ substance withdrawal or other unwanted effects

Index

Note: Page numbers in **bold** refers to tables.

Emergency Triage: Telephone triage and advice, First Edition. Updated version 1.7, 2023.
Edited by Janet Marsden, Mark Newton, Jill Windle and Kevin Mackway-Jones.
© 2016 John Wiley & Sons, Ltd. Published 2016 by John Wiley & Sons, Ltd.

Printed and bound by CPI Group (UK) Ltd, Croydon, CR0 4YY

08/12/2023

08204317-0001